ABOUT THE AUTHOR

Owen O'Kane has dual medical and psychotherapy training and is a former NHS Clinical Lead for Mental Health. His first book *Ten to Zen* was a *Sunday Times* bestseller. Owen lives in London but grew up in Belfast during The Troubles, which he describes as a great training ground for his current work. He also spent many years of his career working with people living with a terminal illness, which has greatly influenced his work. When not writing books, Owen runs his private therapy practice, delivers talks, and contributes to press and media on mental wellness issues. He is a lover of dogs.

Also by Owen O'Kane

Ten to Zen
Ten Times Happier

HOW TO BE YOUR OWN THERAPIST

OWEN O'KANE

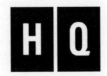

ONE PLACE. MANY STORIES

HQ
An imprint of HarperCollins*Publishers*
1 London Bridge Street
London SE1 9GF

www.harpercollins.co.uk

Harper Ireland
Macken House,
39/40 Mayor Street Upper,
Dublin 1
D01 C9W8

First published in Great Britain by HQ 2022

A catalogue record for this book is available from the British Library.

HB ISBN: 978-0-00-837827-1
TPB ISBN: 978-0-00-859175-5

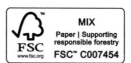

This book is produced from independently certified FSC™ paper
to ensure responsible forest management.

For more information visit: www.harpercollins.co.uk/green

Typeset in Bembo by Palimpsest Book Production Ltd, Falkirk, Stirlingshire

Printed and bound in the UK using 100% renewable electricity
at CPI Group (UK) Ltd

Names, identifying characteristics and details have been changed to protect the
identity and privacy of individuals.

This book is not a substitute for one-to-one live therapy, which some people
will unquestionably need. If you feel you need one-to-one or group
professional support, please prioritise getting help via your doctor or
local mental health organisations. There is a list of support organisations
included at the end of the book.

To my partner Mark, who believed I could
help many people through my books.
Thank you for your belief and encouragement.

CONTENTS

Introduction   1

PART 1

1 What is this therapy malarky?   15
2 What's your story?   33
3 Putting the pieces together   57
4 OK, what now?   84
5 Actions speak louder than words   105

PART 2

6 Get *ready* for your day   131
7 Staying *steady*   159
8 *Reflect and reset* at the end of the day   182
9 When life throws a major curve ball   203
10 All's well that ends well   230

Useful Contact Information   247
Acknowledgements   259

INTRODUCTION

I'm a therapist and, like most therapists, I've been to therapy. It changed my life. In fact, therapy affected me so profoundly that I was inspired to become a therapist myself.

I believe therapy has the potential to change everyone's lives for the better. But here's the problem. It isn't cheap, it's hard to access and there are often waiting lists spanning years. And let's not forget, there's still some degree of stigma attached to therapy! But if you're feeling at all hesitant, consider this: sometimes our brains need a little maintenance and looking after to help us deal with life's challenges. And that's what good therapy helps with. It's nothing weird or freaky. I promise that you won't end up living in a forest or hiding away in a cave. Therapy is for the courageous and what it delivers is true strength and endless possibilities for a fuller life.

After musing on the challenges associated with helping people to get the therapy they need, I had a brainwave. The goal of most therapy is for clients to finish a block of sessions 'skilled up' and 'aware' enough to become their own therapist. So I realised that I needed to write a book that taught people how to do exactly that.

Welcome to *How To Be Your Own Therapist*.

I want this book to be a practical resource that anyone can use. This is not detailed psychoanalysis, and I say that completely unapologetically.

I have the deepest respect for my colleagues who work differently to me, but this isn't a heavyweight academic clinical book. Instead, it aims to simplify complicated theories and make them useable in everyday life. The first half of the book will take you on a personal therapeutic journey, before we get to the daily ten minutes of self-therapy in the second half of the book. We need that first half, otherwise your daily practice won't make any sense. I like to think of the first half as creating a 'new you'; it's like a crash course in therapy, or therapy bootcamp, if you like. The second half is the daily maintenance.

In this book, I will teach you how to access the therapist within you and make the best of each day – whatever is going on for you. The skills you'll learn will help you to function better, feel better and live better for the rest of your life.

One final declaration that might come as a bit of a surprise. *I* am not going to change you. I am offering you my insights, learning and experience. It is *your choice* what you do with it. Too many books, 'gurus' and professionals promise to change your life. I can't do that. But I do believe *you* can change your life.

ABOUT ME

First and foremost, I'm a human being with weaknesses, vulnerabilities and a back catalogue of mistakes like most people. I know from personal experience what it means to be imperfect. I believe this helps a lot in my line of work!

I think we have too many people telling us to do more, be more and buy more, instead of helping us understand how we can live our present lives better and with less struggle. My other bugbear is how often we're told to ignore the warning signs that life is getting on top of us. It's all well and good being told, 'You've got this!' but sometimes we haven't, and we might need a helping hand along the way.

I have a dual medical and psychotherapy background. Before I became a psychotherapist, I was a palliative care specialist. My final job in the NHS was as Clinical Lead for Mental Health in London. I now run my own private therapy practice in London, but I see clients from all over the world. I also deliver talks and workshops internationally on issues related to mental health.

I grew up in Northern Ireland during The Troubles: a period of intense violence between Nationalists and Unionists. It was a challenging childhood. During my own therapy I discovered that, as a result, I was 'hard-wired' to be in a perpetual state of fear, watching out for the next problem. I've since worked on that.

I'm also gay, which meant a lot of interesting conversations while in therapy. Being Irish, Catholic and gay was a conundrum for me. Catholicism in my formative years preached about 'praying the gay away'. So it'll come as no surprise that some of my biggest revelations in therapy were that I tended to consider myself the underdog, and I regularly felt the need to prove my decency as a human being. Therapy taught me I didn't need to prove anything. Instead, I learnt the joy of self-acceptance.

In this book, I will share the personal discoveries

I made about myself with you, to demonstrate what is possible with therapy. I'm talking about break-throughs. Transformation. I am confident you will realise both by reading this book.

HOW DOES THIS BOOK WORK?

THIS BOOK IS DIVIDED INTO TWO PARTS.

Chapters 1 to 5 make up Part 1. This is the essential foundation work that sets you up for your ten minutes of daily therapy practice, which is covered in Part 2. You will need a notebook and a pen to do this work, so be sure you have both ready. Part 1 includes everything you'd usually cover in therapy with me. There are no shortcuts here, so I encourage you to stick with the work. It's life-changing. It will also help you understand the importance of your ten minutes of daily self-therapy. In part 1 we will look at:

1. Your 'real' life story
2. Making sense of your story and how it affects you today
3. What you really want from your life

4. How therapy can help you get what you want
5. The essential ingredients necessary for a more contented life

I'll explain what I mean when I say *your 'real' life story* (since this concept is at the heart of therapy).

It's not simply your recollection of the events of your life in chronological order. What it means is sharing with another person the key events in your life *that mattered to you* and, more importantly, *how they made you feel*. This will include experiences that are positive, negative and everything in between.

Often, we tell ourselves and others versions of our story that are 'rehearsed' or 'respectable', to influence how we want people to see us, as opposed to how we really are. I believe that most people adapt their life stories automatically as a defence mechanism rather than consciously. But personal development and growth only happen when we're able to accept the true events of our past and express them, together with how they made us feel then and how they make us feel now.

That said, it's not enough to just tell your story. Your story also needs to be formulated so that you can connect how and why your experiences have impacted on your emotions, behaviours and ways of thinking today. This will be the second step in your foundation work. Once you're able to do this, everything will become clearer.

We then explore what you want for your future and how to make that future a reality. There is no point doing this work unless it's going to bring some incredible changes to your life. Knowing what you want is crucial, otherwise you may feel directionless.

Making changes to your life so your future looks different from your past will also involve letting go of some of the self-enforced rules you live by that are holding you back. Together, we will work on that.

In the final part of the foundation work, we'll be looking at some essential techniques and self-care tools that you'll be integrating into your ten minutes of daily therapy.

Understanding who you are, why you act as you do, knowing what you want and what to let go of will open the way to a sense of calm, control and clarity.

Chapters 6 to 10 make up Part 2. This half of the book will teach you how to do your ten minutes of daily self-therapy. Here, you'll learn how to integrate techniques learnt in Part 1 into your daily life, and you'll be shown some new ones too. Both will improve your life for the better. This will be your maintenance work. You can do this for as long as you feel you need to. You might feel that you'd benefit from doing some form of this every day indefinitely, making it as much a part of your daily routine as your morning tea or coffee. Your daily therapy is also an opportunity to work on the issues you'll have uncovered while doing the work in Part 1.

Here is a summary of what your daily ten-minute practice will look like, at a glance. I know how demanding life can be, so I've split the ten minutes evenly across your day. This way, no matter how busy you are, you can always make time to check in with yourself. The aim is that these therapy 'boosts' will transform the quality of your day, and ultimately your life!

READY

How long? Four minutes

When? Preferably at the start of your day whenever you can find a gap. I try to think of this time as like brushing my teeth! We all find time to brush our teeth for a few minutes at the start of the day, so why shouldn't we prioritise our mental wellness in the same way?

What's it for? Quietening the chatter inside your head and shifting your mindset into a more flexible, adaptive place that helps you get the most out of your day.

STEADY

How long? Three minutes

When? After you've had your lunch.

What's it for? Keeping you steady for the day and managing any setbacks that may have taken place. Regulating how you think and react, and ensuring you psychologically look after yourself as the day progresses.

REFLECT AND RESET

How long? Three minutes

When? Just before you go to bed, you're comfortable, you have nothing more to do and you're undistracted by your phone.

What's it for? Exploring the lessons from the day and letting go of unhelpful thoughts to enable a full night's sleep.

The ten minutes of daily self-therapy I teach you in this book will be life-affirming, and transformative. They will also be a time when your entire self will be acknowledged and accepted with compassion. Having said that, some of the questions, exercises and suggestions in this book will be taking you outside of your comfort zone. That's unavoidable. Therapy *should* get under your skin (in a good way). But here's the deal: it works. Think of it as a decluttering exercise for your mind, to help you function better.

Different therapists have different approaches, and I am going to teach you how to perform self-therapy in a very particular way, a way that other therapists might not. In short, the views in this book are mine. What I teach here is not representative of the views of any one professional or regulatory body. Instead, the work I'll be taking you through in this book takes an integrative approach based on my various trainings and personal experiences, and from knowing what works in clinical practice. It's also informed by a range of therapy models rather than one single model (although I've taken care not to get too technical and stick with straightforward language). This integrative therapeutic approach will, I hope, bring ease and a sense of stability.

For interest, models of therapy used here include Cognitive Behavioural Therapy (CBT), Compassion Focused Therapy (CFT), Mindfulness, and Interpersonal Psychotherapy. For anyone with a particular interest in different therapy models, there's a lot of useful information online, particularly on the websites of professional therapy organisations such as www.bps.org.uk.

I will explain fully every part of the process as I

guide you through it, in order, and I promise I'll avoid jargon, clichés and psychobabble as much as I can. I am asking you to trust me, even in the moments when the questions I'm asking you may not make much sense, or if the process of doing the work makes you feel lousy. Therapy can be tough, but it should never overwhelm you. Work at a pace that's comfortable for you and remember, there's no rush. You have the rest of your life to work on this.

A FINAL NOTE BEFORE WE BEGIN

Throughout this book, I will share case studies aimed to provide support and help. It is for adults looking for a self-directed set of therapy tools to get the best from their day, their life and themselves. It is also for teenagers with the support from their parents. Wherever you are at, it will help. But it's not a substitute for one-to-one live therapy, which some people will unquestionably need. If you do feel you need one-to-one or group professional support, please prioritise getting help via your doctor or local mental health organisations. There is a list of support organisations included at the end of the book.

Please also be mindful that it would not be sensible

to engage with this work if you are feeling very overwhelmed, experiencing psychotic symptoms, feeling suicidal or don't have adequate support around you. You will need professional help in these circumstances.

It is also not advisable to engage with this work if you are under the influence of alcohol, drugs or any other unprescribed substances.

Finally, all names, details and case studies featured in this book have been changed, and any individuals or organisations mentioned have been anonymised, to protect and respect client confidentiality.

PART 1

CHAPTER 1

WHAT IS THIS THERAPY MALARKY?

I'm going to teach you to become your own therapist and make therapy part of your life for ten minutes every day. But before I do that, I'd like to talk about the shame and stigma surrounding therapy.

I'm always intrigued when I meet a new client who says to me at the end of a session, 'Wow, that wasn't so bad.' (It's usually men.) I always ask what they mean, as the preconceptions surrounding therapy fascinate me and, as you might expect, I've heard a range of responses back. Brace yourself!

'You seem like a normal guy for a
  therapist.'
'It wasn't as weird as I expected.'
'I'm surprised we laughed.'
'It wasn't all, "How did that make you
  feel?"'
'You didn't seem shocked by what I said.'
'You didn't hypnotise me.'
'I thought you would just nod your head and
  say, "I understand."'
'It made more sense than I expected.'
'It wasn't all tears and feelings.'
'I was expecting you to be a tw*t.' (And
  variations on that theme.)

It doesn't stop there. I sometimes avoid telling people in social settings what I do for a living. I find my occupation often either worries people (they think I'm mind-reading or 'diagnosing' them based on our small talk), or makes them feel the need to disclose their entire life story, or it freaks them out.

When I worked as a clinical lead for an NHS therapy service, I learnt that some words associated with mental health stopped people attending groups. For example, if we set up a group called 'Coping with Depression', it would be empty. If we set up a group called 'Boost Your Mood', it would be full.

I work with clients who ask me to remove the word 'therapist' from the invoice. I have even been asked to remove my title from the office door. Some patients are concerned about what others might think if they knew they were seeing a therapist. A medical doctor specialising in the body rather than the mind would be unlikely to get the same request, unless it was in an area like sexual health. Therapists seem to be something of a 'dirty secret'.

I remember going for my first therapy session in my early twenties (a few years ago now), sneaking up the road, terrified someone would see me. I had the look of someone engaging in an illicit affair. Luckily my first therapist was a nun, dispelling any such potential rumours. Her office was in a convent. I was relieved when I discovered this because it was a useful cover-up. I could be at a confession of sorts!

Being serious, though, I was ashamed that I needed help. I was ashamed that I couldn't work it out alone. I was concerned what others would think of me. I was ashamed I was struggling mentally with 'coming out'. This was complicated further with a cultural belief at the time, a belief which I'd internalised, that men don't struggle. Boys don't cry.

Which brings me to this. *A lot of people consider it shameful to need therapy.* I used to be one of those people! There is *still* a degree of stigma around mental ill health. Making the responsible choice to be in therapy is *still* considered a sign of weakness or a failing. Likewise, therapists and therapy are *still* quite mysterious to some people. Sadly, these negative preconceptions are mostly driven by fear. Public perception of therapy is a lot more positive now than it was one or two decades ago. More people *are* coming forward for help. But that stigma is still very much around.

If you're feeling even a hint of this discomfort and anxiety I'm talking about, please let me help allay any nervousness you might have right now.

The truth is, despite the ongoing shame around it, every single person on the planet would benefit from some therapy. Even if you're perfectly content with your life, gaining the self-knowledge to understand *why* you're happy means you can re-discover what makes you tick when life is less than rosy. Everyone, no matter how wonderful their life might seem from the outside, will experience some seriously tough times, and it's not easy navigating those ups and downs. Sometimes we need support. That's why in this book, you will learn:

- What therapy does to your brain, and how it helps, in a nutshell
- The process of therapy in more detail
- What you'll be doing in self-therapy

WHAT THERAPY DOES TO YOUR BRAIN, AND HOW IT HELPS, IN A NUTSHELL

I have worked for thirty years with people in distress. And what I've learnt in that time is that it's the *response* to a negative experience, rather than the experience itself, that has the biggest psychological impact. Some people cope well and adjust to horrible experiences. Some people suffer deeply.

I don't believe people choose to suffer. I believe some people are programmed to suffer more than others, or get stuck in unhelpful patterns of behaviour.

How much a person suffers because of their response to negative experiences could be linked to how they think, how they deal with emotions, what rules they have in place for their life or how they behave. Most of these patterns are learnt or inherited as children and then carried into adulthood. You will learn more about this later.

In essence, a lot of adults are going through life using childhood coping strategies. And that, in my experience, is the root of much human distress.

The good news is therapy can change that, as thousands of research papers can attest to. Therapy means standing outside of your life and having a look inside, but doing so objectively. You can make fascinating discoveries about yourself when you play the formative events of your life back and begin to understand why you struggle. Therapy will encourage you to tell your life story and connect your experiences to what you struggle with today. It will help you understand patterns of thought, automated emotional responses, why you behave as you do and how you can change what keeps you stuck.

Each day in my practice I see people trying to manage issues such as anxiety, depression, trauma, loss, relationship issues and conflict. Therapy helps them unravel the cause of their pain and offers guidance that can ease their suffering. It is a collaborative process rather than a prescriptive one.

The joy of modern therapy is that it uses strategies informed by the latest cutting-edge research in medicine, neuroscience, social sciences and pharmacology. That is to say, we are complex physical, emotional, thinking beings, and we need more than psychological insights to help us function at our best. Good therapy should always be holistic in its approach, by which I mean it should consider the whole person.

LET'S LOOK AT THE FACTS ABOUT THERAPY:

1. It is a scientifically proven method of improving mental wellness
2. It improves brain chemistry
3. It can reprogram neuropathways to help a person function in more helpful ways
4. It improves quality of life
5. It improves mood and anxiety issues
6. It improves work life, home life and general motivation
7. It helps people break the cycle of destructive behavioural patterns
8. It eases distress

THE PROCESS OF THERAPY: UNDERSTANDING THE MECHANICS IN MORE DETAIL

As I mentioned, I'm going to give you a therapy crash course. Think of it like a compressed version of the work I would ordinarily do with a client. This foundation work is essential. Then we'll move on to the maintenance work: the ten minutes a day of self-therapy. I've deliberately chosen ten minutes, partly because quick acts of self-care can fit more easily into busy schedules, but also because you've a better chance of committing to the self-therapy long term if it's a much more achievable ten minutes, as opposed to an hour.

I want to explain the basics of how therapy works by using the analogy of a cake with three layers.

The processes I explain here will come alive when you are doing the actual work. For now, though, I hope this analogy will offer some insight into why I suggest the exercises I do. Just know that if I am suggesting you try something, there will be a strong clinical reason for doing so – we'll cover that in more detail shortly.

The top layer of the cake is your thoughts and feelings. Your thoughts and your feelings are separate but interconnected, and they're constantly communicating with each other. For example, if the rather unwelcome thought, 'My partner doesn't care about me,' crops up in your mind, it will automatically create a feeling of sadness or something similar.

Likewise, you may experience a sudden shift in your emotional state that leads to a catalogue of unhelpful thoughts. When you are sad, it may prove difficult to have optimistic thoughts about yourself or your life. Thoughts may sound more like, 'I'm not good enough,' 'I'm a disappointment' or 'I'm rubbish.'

Thinking is a cognitive process. Sometimes it's automated and unconscious. You could be working and suddenly your mind jumps to a memory of a holiday. Sometimes it's conscious. For example, you might be wondering what to buy at the supermarket, or the best route to a wedding next weekend, or considering how to proceed with a delicate contractual negotiation. Thoughts come with a narrative, with one thought often leading to another.

An emotion, on the other hand, is an automated (that is to say, automatic) experience that you *feel*. Thoughts may or may not be attached. It may be in response to an event. It may happen unexpectedly. Our emotions are like the weather, they can fluctuate between two extremes in a very short space of time. Learning to acknowledge them and letting them guide you is key.

Neuroscientists estimate that we have between 60,000 to 80,000 thoughts a day! That explains the expression 'a mind in overdrive'! We are thinking all the time. But thinking itself isn't the problem.

The problem is that critical, catastrophic or inflexible ways of thinking, and negative emotional responses, often become automatic. We've learnt them from our early life experiences. For example, if someone comes from a family with very critical parents, they may automatically think the worst of themselves and struggle with negative thoughts when they are in situations that mirror aspects of their childhood. Consequently, regulating emotions may prove a problem.

By that same token, someone could have learnt as a child that some emotions aren't acceptable, such as anger, fear or vulnerability. They may struggle as an adult dealing with these emotions, and consequently experience negative thought patterns whenever these emotions arise.

I've worked with many clients who weren't given permission to show vulnerability as children. When they are in situations that evoke difficult-to-handle emotions as an adult, they automatically have very critical thoughts about themselves, such as, 'I shouldn't be feeling this way,' 'I am weak' or 'I am useless.' In short, they have been programmed to respond in a particular way in certain scenarios due to their early life experiences.

Automated thinking and emotional responses tend to be habitual. Unless, of course, we stop to evaluate how they are negatively impacting our life and make a conscious effort to change our responses. Therapy brings hope here. New ways of thinking and healthier emotional responses can be opted for. Change is possible.

But good therapy won't just focus on the top layer

of the cake. Sure, that's fine for a quick fix in the emotions and thoughts department. But if you want the secret to *long-lasting* change? You need to look at those middle and bottom layers too, as both these layers directly impact our thoughts and feelings.

Let's look at that middle layer. This one's interesting. It's the rules and beliefs that we inherit from families, culture, religion, gender and every formative experience we have. It dictates (either consciously or subconsciously) how we think we ought to be living our lives. It's less visible than the top layer, and more ingrained.

We learn very early in life that if we're going to fit in, belong, be safe, be taken seriously, be accepted, and so on, we need to 'play the game'. Playing the game means sticking with our inherited rules and beliefs. These are the prerequisites for acceptance into society, or so we're led to believe. These prerequisites will look different for every person, depending on their situation. But the ones that I see crop up again and again are perfection, success, reliability, selflessness, being a good person, being in control and being emotionally 'strong'. I also hear lots of clients talk about how important it is that they're not considered needy, weak, vulnerable, opinionated, a failure or a disappointment.

In theory, there is nothing wrong with having

rules and beliefs around what constitutes 'functioning well' in life, especially if they work and don't cause distress. The middle layer of the cake is an important part of the structure after all. But the problem is, rules and beliefs are often inflexible. And inflexibility is a difficult force to reckon with.

If your personal rules dictate that you *must* be perfect, good, successful and so on, then life will be a challenge. No one can be all of those things all of the time. Likewise, if you believe it is your duty to please people, that you should *never* disappoint others, *always* be the best and so on, then life will be a challenge. You are human. Rigid, inflexible rules and beliefs will cause distress, which will manifest in negative thoughts and emotions.

Think of a time when you told yourself that you had to be perfect at something, and it didn't go to plan. If you have (or had, at the time) inflexible beliefs around perfectionism, then the outcome may have, predictably, been negative, self-critical or self-deprecating thoughts. Your emotions will have been dominated by a sense of not being good enough, of having failed or disappointed others. Your rules and beliefs will have created a thought and emotion distress response.

On the other hand, if you were to have had a more flexible approach to your rules and beliefs, then the scenario could have played out differently. An imperfect outcome can be managed with compassionate thoughts, for example, 'I did my best and I can learn from this for next time.' Emotionally, that's easier to manage.

Put simply, reviewing, adapting and creating more flexibility with your rules and beliefs will help you unlearn negative automated thoughts and emotions. Therapy can help with this.

Let's do a quick recap before we move on to the bottom layer of the cake, which is even more interesting.

The top layer of the cake is our thoughts and emotions, which are inextricably connected. These thoughts and emotions are directly affected by the second layer, our rules and beliefs.

On to the third layer. You won't be surprised to hear that this one influences everything. This is the epicentre of therapy. Our deeper *foundation core beliefs*.

Different models of therapy will explain this in different ways, but the meaning is the same. Foundation core beliefs are the foundations upon which your entire world view and psychological make-up are based. They can be divided into four main categories and this is how they normally present:

- **Safety and security:** Either a belief that you are safe, or a belief that you are not safe
- **Lovability:** Either a belief that you are lovable, or a belief that you are not lovable
- **Self-worth:** Either a belief that you have value, or a belief that you do not have value
- **Hope:** Either feeling hopeful, or feeling hopeless

Let's look at an example. If someone never felt safe or loved as a child, this will influence their belief systems. Rules and beliefs will be focused on staying safe: I must not take risks, I must have a plan, I must have certainty. I should please people, or they may reject me. I must never show vulnerability, or I could be abandoned.

Consequently, this person may also have difficulty with negative or critical patterns of thinking and find managing their emotions challenging. Their life experience has created foundational core beliefs that lead to an unsteady bedrock. This is played out in how the person thinks, feels and reacts to everyday life. None of it is their fault and this is also something therapy seeks to address, in that it not only tackles the primary problems but also any secondary self-blaming or shaming.

WHAT YOU'LL BE DOING IN SELF-THERAPY

Most people think therapy is going along for a weekly chat, reflecting on life, and hopefully making improvements to their mental wellbeing in order to have a more enjoyable life. If that's what you're looking for, this book may not be right for you. I think it's best we clear that up straight away.

In my experience, most people won't have break-throughs unless therapy is an active, collaborative process. For me, talking is just one part of therapy. It is also:

- Working between sessions
- A series of actions, not just words, e.g. changes in behaviour
- Creating a new model of self-care that teaches you to look after yourself
- Committing to the process as an ongoing way of life
- Working with the connections between mind–body emotions
- A willingness to be challenged
- A willingness to let go of old patterns
- Not expecting the therapist to do all the work

- A willingness to be curious and open to a process full of possibilities
- A willingness to change

I'd like to explain why certain strategies that I'll be encouraging you to use in your self-therapy are helpful:

Recounting or reflecting on your life: this helps you process your experiences (and by 'process', I mean, 'allowing your brain to acknowledge what's happened and file your memories away in the appropriate place in your brain').

Action-based activities: consolidates what you know and helps change behaviours or patterns.

Writing things down: makes you more likely to action the changes that are needed.

Challenging patterns of thought: creates more helpful ways of thinking that will serve you better.

Regulating emotions: gets you comfortable with all your humanity and prevents you from getting trapped with repressed emotions.

Accepting uncomfortable truths: chances are, I'll have heard several versions of what you're describing before, and I'll have learnt a few things that tend to be true when it comes to the situation you're describing. They can be hard to hear, but it's so important to face up to uncomfortable truths if you want to move forward.

As I hope you will discover in your therapy journey, therapy is active, not passive. It's about how you live, how you move, how you breathe, how you think, how you deal with life, how you react, how you care for yourself, how you treat yourself.

It's getting to know yourself. It's telling your story. It's understanding your story. It's knowing what you want. It's also knowing what you must do to make the changes you need. It's a revamp of your life.

WHAT'S REQUIRED OF YOU?

I'm going to keep this section short and sweet.

All I ask of you is that you turn up, keep an open mind, trust the process and put the work in. Above all, don't give yourself a hard time.

If you feel you need more help than this book can offer, don't hesitate to stop, and speak to your doctor or a professional.

Shall we get started? I'd like to know a little more about you.

CHAPTER 2

WHAT'S YOUR STORY?

Everyone experiences hard times, no matter how perfect their life might look.

As children, when life gets tough, we can avoid everyday responsibilities and healthily escape into our own heads more easily than we can as adults. But when we reach adulthood, we're forced to deal with life in all its rawness, and with all the (often painful!) awareness and insight that this stage of our life brings.

Many years ago I lived in Dublin, and 'What's the story?' was a common greeting, in place of 'Hello' or 'How's it going?' Of course, no one ever expected a full blow-by-blow account of whatever your story was that day. But it was polite to ask all the same. I love this greeting because it shows a genuine interest in the other person, or at least an acknowledgement of their story in that moment.

Today I ask a similar question: 'What's your story?' Your story will have many hidden treasures that help you understand who you are and how you can live a fuller life.

Threaded throughout your story will be darkness and light, failure and success, loss and redemption, hopelessness and hope. All are part of life's rich tapestry. But the problem is that the tougher experiences stick to us like glue and longer term can create mood fluctuations, anxiety and issues with our day-to-day functioning.

I want to teach you how to handle these challenges and navigate your way around life's everyday ups and downs using daily self-therapy.

But before I embark upon the journey of teaching you to become your own therapist, we need to do the groundwork. I know it's a pain and you might be thinking, 'Just give me the solutions.' But the truth is, *you* are the solution, which is why we need to start with your story. *Because your story matters and it's worth telling.*

Telling your story will help you connect what went on in your life with the person you are today. The events of your life are like the pieces of a jigsaw puzzle. As you begin to fit the pieces together, you eventually reach a point where you can see the whole picture. That whole picture represents all there is to know about who you are, and why you are that way. For example, a child who has been left alone a lot by their parents may develop a fear of abandonment in adulthood. The self-awareness that comes from telling your story – putting together the pieces of the jigsaw – is the essence of therapy. That self-awareness will help you feel safer, calmer and more at ease when you're feeling down, or scared, or out of control. It will also help you bounce back quicker.

The story of your life will lead you to your 'Aha!' moments. These are moments of sudden insight. Believe it or not, your story is your power. While you can't change it, you can salvage strength and wisdom from it. All of it, even the messy parts. I believe no therapy or self-help can truly help you until you come to terms with your story and accept it for what it is rather than what you wanted it to be.

But that's not enough. It's also important to tell your story to other people. That's where the empowerment lies. When you find the courage to tell your story, you are also saying that you are no longer ashamed of it. And that's life-changing.

So I'd love to invite you, maybe for the first time ever, to tell your story.

A CAUTIONARY NOTE

Before we get into the nitty gritty of this part of the process, you will likely have tried-and-tested methods of dealing with questions around your life. Maybe you have a selection of rehearsed versions of your story, each serving a different purpose, that you roll out as the situation requires.

It might be that you unconsciously employ some clever psychological tricks to either avoid telling your story or to change it to something more acceptable or appropriate:

Denial, where you don't want to accept what's happened to you. This might sound like, 'It was all OK.'

Minimising, where you downplay an experience that had a significant effect on you in order to avoid the pain caused by that experience. This might sound like, 'I guess it could have been worse.'

Catastrophising, where you exaggerate the negative aspects of your experience because you need your suffering to be acknowledged by someone else. This might sound like, 'It was all awful.'

Ruminating, where you (mistakenly) believe that the more you think about aspects of your story, the more it'll help you. This might sound like, 'There was this time and another time, and then this other time . . .'

Dissociation, where you treat your story as if it were someone else's, or refuse to engage with it to avoid the pain caused by your story. This might sound like, 'I don't remember much.'

Avoidance, where it's easier for you to avoid talking about your story as it makes you uneasy. This might sound like, 'I don't like talking about this.'

Fantasising, where you want to pretend either that something happened in your life that didn't, or that something didn't happen in your life that did. This might sound like, 'It was all absolutely wonderful.'

Repressing, where you bury a memory in the hope that it will go away. This might sound like, 'I'd rather focus on the future and not talk about this.'

If you feel yourself falling into the trap of employing these tricks or telling the rehearsed versions of your story, gently stop wherever you are during the process, rewind, then start your story again without judgement.

When I first went to therapy in my early twenties, I thought I was pretty 'sorted'. It might even have appeared that way to those around me. I was about to come out as gay and I thought talking to someone beforehand seemed like a sensible idea. In the first session, I started to tell my story to the therapist in a very mechanical, rehearsed way. It was all fine. I was fine. My life was fine. My family were fine. Everything was fine, fine, fine! The therapist paused and very calmly, said to me, 'You tell me you're fine, but you look a little sad.' And that was the end of being fine. I suddenly found myself crying and we started the session again. Of course, I wasn't fine, and it was time to stop pretending. Not only was this a relief but it was also the beginning of a new understanding of myself that I would never have discovered alone. Who would have thought Mr Fine had got it so wrong for so many years?

WHERE DO I START?

This is a common question when I ask clients to tell me their story. First of all, I never ask for a detailed account of someone's life because I believe it can encourage rumination (deep thinking that can keep us stuck). Instead, I prefer a movie trailer version simply because I get more focus and less digression that way.

This 'movie trailer version' is achieved by a process called a **timeline**, which happens in four stages:

1. **Writing a first draft of your timeline (i.e. your life story)**
2. **Second edition: the rewrite**
3. **Third edition: how did that feel?**
4. **Sharing your story with someone who will respect its richness**

This structure will help you stay focused on the important aspects of your story and hopefully make this a cathartic experience for you. I am encouraging you to tell your story in a new way so that you can begin to assess it rationally from the outside. Sometimes we can get so emotionally invested in the way we're telling our story, rather than the story itself, that we can't step back and assess what's happened in a balanced, logical way. Likewise, it's not uncommon to completely disconnect from your story or talk about it as if it happened to someone else.

I once treated a 21-year-old client who, when I asked them to write their timeline, returned with a blank page saying they couldn't recall anything in their life worth recording. While I was aware this wasn't true, the blank page indicated that there was a lot to work on here, and it acted as a good starting point. A way in. It truly represented the sense of emptiness and disconnection they felt when they thought about their life.

However, unlike this client, *you're* being your own therapist here, so it's important that you invest time in doing the work. This part of the process is where the gold is, so the more effort you put in, the more you'll get out of it.

STAGE 1

WRITING A FIRST DRAFT OF YOUR TIMELINE (I.E. YOUR LIFE STORY)

The only person qualified to write your story is you. No one else can accurately describe what it has been like to live your life. While other people may be able to talk about the events of your life that they're aware of, no one else knows about all the private conversations, the quiet shared moments, or even which events have had the biggest impact on you. You are the expert on your story, so it needs to be told by you, and you alone, completely unedited, warts and all.

It's entirely your decision how you decide to capture your story. Most people opt to write it down, but over the years I've seen drawings, paintings, poetry, songs and even a mini film! It doesn't matter which method you choose. The important point is that the story gets told.

When recollecting the events of your life, I suggest you block out a few hours and go somewhere private where you won't be interrupted. Try to consider this exercise as an important event, almost like turning up for a big meeting that could have life-changing consequences. I suggest you choose a place that is comfortable and calming for you. Don't try to do this while the dog is jumping on you or when you're cooking dinner. This is your opportunity to carry out a piece of work that could have a powerful, positive impact on your life. You need to give it your undivided time and attention.

If at any point while you're writing down your story it becomes too distressing, then you can stop for a break and come back when you're ready. If you have concerns that it is simply going to be too difficult to do alone then you can always seek the guidance of a professional therapist. While the process may be uncomfortable in parts, it's worth considering that anything worthwhile is rarely easy.

As I am guiding you through the process, I am going to use the writing method, but you can amend as needed if you decide to go down one of the other routes.

How about an example before we start? Let's say you're 40 years old. You want to be reflecting over all the key events in your life to date, from infancy to the present. I suggest you approach the timeline in blocks of about ten years. For example, ages 0-9, 10-19, 20-29 and 30-40.

If you are unable to recall specific memories from a young age, that's OK. There may be family stories that involve you, but if you can't recall the memory, don't force it. This must be *your* account.

Here's an example of what a timeline might look like:

Age/ Year	Experience Health, family, education/job, significant life events, etc.	Meaning What it meant to me at the time (e.g. I was alone, unloved, unfairly treated; others hurt me, rejected me.)
0–9		
10–19		
20–29		
30–40		

First, you're going to list all the happy, joyful, cele-bratory or positive events and periods in your life at the top of each box. This might be winning an award, the beginning of a new relationship and falling in love, landing a job or doing well in an exam, a wonderful holiday, a time when all your hard work paid off, an amazing party - anything that felt life-affirming. I strongly encourage you not to overthink or analyse what comes up. Simply allow the memory to surface and jot it down without judgement. Non-judgement and honesty are key here.

In a separate box you're going to do the same thing, but this time focusing on the sad, difficult and negative memories. This could be a break-up, a bereavement, losing a job, failing at something, being bullied, illness, or something you're ashamed of having done. Inevitably, you'll be revisiting some uncomfortable memories that will make this part of the process more difficult. This is 100 per cent normal, so please try not to panic if it doesn't 'feel good'. Therapy can be challenging. Allowing yourself to access some of the darker parts of your experience will lead to growth. Or, as I sometimes like to say, crops can't grow without crap!

Whether a negative or positive memory, keep in mind that other people's opinions don't matter. For instance, if a memory comes up that, for whatever reason evokes particular associations, perhaps you were sad when a younger sibling came along, or happy when a mean grandparent died, note it down. Allow it to be as it is, and not how you think others think it should be.

STAGE 2

SECOND EDITION: THE REWRITE

Once you've completed your first draft, I suggest you step away from the timeline for a day or two. Your brain will be processing all the old memories you've dredged to the surface, and some new ones might emerge.

After you've taken a couple of days, reread your timeline with these questions in mind:

- Does this read as a true, raw, authentic version of my story?
- Does it capture the moments of struggle and pain?
- Have I sugar-coated some of the details or left events out?
- Have I been brutally honest with myself?

Are these questions making you reconsider what you've written? Are there any memories you missed the first time around or any gaps you need to fill? Does the order of events need tweaking? If so, feel free to edit your timeline (bearing in mind, before you do, that it's also fine to keep hold of a copy of your original timeline, if you'd like to. It might be interesting to see how the story has changed.)

If some of your reflections don't fit neatly into the timeline, make a separate set of notes and put them in a safe place to revisit if you need to.

STAGE 3

THIRD EDITION: HOW DID THAT FEEL?

So far, we've focused on the details of your story. But this is about learning to become your own therapist. So – you knew it was coming! – we need to talk about those tricky feelings, too.

Before we go any further, I want to add a note here about feelings. Many of us think that we should be experiencing 'positive' feelings all the time, and that 'negative' feelings are a sign that something's wrong. This is partly because good feelings feel better and partly because we're constantly being told that we should have a positive mindset by social, online and print media and commercial advertisers. But feeling good isn't possible all the time, because a life lived fully will always have difficult periods with plenty of negative emotions and moments upon which we can reflect and learn. And these negative emotions serve a purpose, just as your positive emotions do. In fact, I like to think of our feelings as barometers, signposts back to steadiness. Life is a mixed bag of emotional experiences and that's how it's supposed to be. How can we appreciate the good times if we have no experience of the tough times?

In short, *all* emotions are trying to help and guide you. Rather than categorise them as 'good' and 'bad', instead try to welcome them and see them as interesting. It's incredibly liberating.

Let's bring this back to your timeline. It's worth pondering what feelings came up for you when you reflected on the events in the story of your life – both the first and the second edition. Perhaps some reactions surprised you or maybe there were moments when you didn't feel what you expected to feel. Keep a note, maybe with a different colour pen, of the feelings that emerged when recalling your important life events. I encourage you to be curious about this array of emotions that will surround the important points of your life. If you can't access these emotions for whatever reason, that's OK, so long as it helps you realise something about yourself – perhaps that you disconnect from certain feelings. Or maybe it's hard to label some of your feelings, which is OK too, but that's something worth working on.

Remember, at this stage you're not trying to do anything with the feelings, you're just discovering what's there and allowing yourself to feel. Underneath the feeling there might be some new information or an 'Aha!' moment. But don't try to force it, just allow it to come naturally.

I remember doing this exercise in my own therapy and uncovering something interesting. I recalled a memory as a young teenager when I got homesick on a school trip. I was very upset about being away from home, and this meant that a teacher had to drive me back to my parents. When I explored my emotions surrounding this event, I noticed that I felt embarrassed and ashamed when I'd previously thought I had just been anxious about being away. These emotions taught me my concern was about disappointing my parents, leading to a sense of embarrassment and shame. Fast forward a few years and I realised that this one seemingly trivial event contributed to me developing a belief that I needed to always see things through to avoid embarrassment or shame.

It's fascinating what these feelings can teach us if we allow them to. We will talk more about what you can learn from your emotional responses to past events in Chapter 3 when we roadmap your story. But for now, being aware of the feelings, and asking the question, 'I wonder what that's about?' are enough. The awareness will come.

I strongly discourage you from over-thinking, over-analysing or excessively ruminating on the events of the past, or your emotional responses, during this exercise. Some memories will hold more weight than others. Some reactions won't make sense. A happy memory might evoke a sad emotion. A difficult memory might evoke a series of emotions or even a sense of numbness. There is no right or wrong response. Your emotions are what they are. But they will teach you something about who you are and how you respond to life. I can guarantee that.

Alongside documenting your responses to specific past events, it might also be useful to reflect on how the overall experience of devising your timeline made you feel. Here are some common responses I often hear:

- I thoroughly enjoyed it
- It was tough
- I tried to avoid it
- I kept putting it off
- I was keen to finish it quickly

- I was hoping to avoid my past
- It was incredibly surprising
- I had buried so many memories
- I had forgotten many of the nice times
- It was emotional

Your experience of sitting down to create your timeline can be as revealing as your emotional responses to events. So you know, I felt a little irritated when I did mine because I was facing aspects of my life I had avoided for a long time. The irritation told me much about my avoidance. I realised I sometimes try to dodge facing up to the uncomfortable stuff in my life.

Your own feelings during this exercise may not make as much sense to you right now, and that's completely OK. We're going to work on that part of the process in Chapter 3 when you 'map out' your story and link it to your current life.

STAGE 4

SHARING YOUR STORY WITH SOMEONE WHO WILL RESPECT ITS RICHNESS

There is an expression, 'everyone has a book in them.' And I believe this is true. Everyone has a story to tell that is completely unique to them. And I think it's deeply important that everyone has an opportunity to tell their story. When you tell your story, you are seen, heard and hopefully validated.

I worked in palliative care for many years and I would occasionally meet people close to death who'd never had the opportunity to tell their story. Sometimes, they would share it with me. These moments were golden. It was a privilege to listen. Watching their eyes brighten and dim as they journeyed through their life was incredibly moving. I've lost count of the number of times I've heard a dying person say:

- It's a relief to tell someone this
- I'm glad someone knows this
- Thanks for listening to me
- I didn't think anyone would be interested in my story
- I feel like a weight has been lifted

And that sense of a weight being lifted was tangible with almost every story.

You have an opportunity now to tell your story in all its fullness and glory while you're alive. You don't have to wait until the end of your life, or worse, never tell your story at all. And the time is now because ultimately now is all we have. Tomorrow is guaranteed to no one.

HOW TO TELL YOUR STORY

I'm going to avoid being overly prescriptive here because *you* will know how to tell your story best, simply because it's yours. There is no person better placed than you.

All I'm going to do here is share a few tips that should help you get as much as possible out of this experience.

First, choose someone you're comfortable with. Explain to them that you have been creating a timeline of your life. When I'm working with a client, I always suggest they find someone they consider a genuine **pal**. They are usually someone who is:

P: Present

A: Accepting

L: Loving

Avoid the friend or family member that interrupts, judges, interjects with their own stories or shows any sign of disrespect for your story.

I will say here that if any of the content of your story is highly distressing or traumatic, please don't hesitate to seek advice from your doctor or a mental health professional. Most issues can be handled within personal networks, but it is good to be mindful that sometimes professional interventions are important and essential.

Find a location that's quiet and private. A pub or nightclub may not be the best choice for this one! Then it's over to you. Share your timeline with someone and give them the gift of your story unapologetically and honestly. Remember, you are showing up, lowering your defences and letting someone see you *as you truly are*, without any of the social armour we all use to protect us. This takes enormous courage. You are courageous.

As you tell your story, try to avoid digressing or allowing the listener to 'therapise' you as you talk. Allow the story to flow naturally. Let the emotions rise, pause when you need to, breathe, smile, cry and take pride in your steps towards transformation.

When this part of the work is completed, the next step is salvaging what you can from your story. This is the 'mapping out' stage and the beginning of what will, in time, develop into a much fuller understanding of who you are and why you are this way. More on this in Chapter 3.

For now, I leave you to tell your story.

NIGEL'S STORY

I find it useful to share case studies because I think they often bring issues to life or clarify questions you might have.

Nigel worked for a large corporation. He arrived at my office seeking support with three issues:

- Anxiety (often heightened on Sunday evenings)
- Relationship difficulties
- Feeling a sense of failure

None of his issues made sense to him. He was good at his job, interpersonally warm and had a hugely successful career. He angrily blurted out, 'I just don't understand any of these bullsh*t feelings!' I was confident we could make sense of it, and I assured him of that.

After the initial introductory session, we explored his timeline, which he resented doing. He said he felt irritated as he wanted therapy to make him 'happy', not upset. But naturally, the timeline was instrumental in helping us make sense of his struggle.

He came from a loving family who did their best by him, and he didn't identify any major traumas in his life. There were of course highs and lows, heart-aches, break-ups and some difficult times. However, one key period in his life generated a huge reaction on his timeline.

Nigel was sent to private school aged 11. His parents believed it would be good for him, but he was unhappy as his friends had gone to school locally. He never told them as he feared they would be disappointed. He wanted to go to a drama school, but knew it wasn't something his parents wanted for him. It set in motion a sense of failure.

He recounted a sense of dread he always felt on Sundays. This Sunday-night dread never left, and it was during therapy we discovered that his corporate job was an extension of school. He didn't want to be there, and he wasn't living the life he wanted. His anxiety was now making sense to him.

Nigel also discovered that he'd felt unheard when he was sent to private school. As an adult he could see his parents were doing what they thought was best for him, but as a teenager he'd felt unheard by them. This had led to Nigel being mistrustful of people who wanted to get close to him. He described deliberately sabotaging a romantic relationship to avoid rejection. This mistrust in people had never been resolved.

If Nigel hadn't found the courage to tell his story, we would never have figured out the core reason behind his struggles. His anxiety, relationship issues and feelings of failure all made perfect sense now. Nigel was subsequently able to focus on unlearning his unhelpful beliefs around trust, himself and other people.

CHAPTER 3

PUTTING THE PIECES TOGETHER

I've used this metaphor before but I'm going to roll it out again, since I think it explains the point I need to make here perfectly: therapy can be a little like doing a jigsaw. There are many pieces – that is, the main highs and lows of your life. But the full picture – all there is to know about who you are, and why you are that way – isn't clear until they are all put together. A jigsaw with a missing piece will always be incomplete. We need all the pieces.

It's the same when working through the parts of our story. We can't pick and choose which experiences to focus on because they feel good. If we are to understand who we are and why we are that way, we need to understand our whole story, even if that means confronting some ugly feelings, or times when we might have behaved badly or been made to feel small.

You might be wondering why understanding your story is so important. It's all in the past, after all. I've lost count of the number of times I've heard, 'Do I really have to go through all this?' in the therapy room. And the short answer is yes! Because within your story there are gems of information that will help create life-changing awareness in your life now. Your story has more power than you might think.

I've also said this before but it's worth saying again: no one else can recount your story or make sense of it the way you can. I can provide the guidance, but you are the expert of your life. I often remind my clients of this. I can never really know how a client feels or has experienced a life event. Yes, I can hypothesise and empathise, but I can never truly go through what they went through.

This reminds me of a therapy client, Julie, who recounted a painful memory of not getting new shoes on the first day of school, aged 10. All the other children appeared to have new shoes and she didn't. At the time, her family was struggling financially and her dad was dependent on alcohol. As she told this story, she wept inconsolably. As I watched her cry, I assumed her upset was linked to embarrassment or other shame-related feelings around her school friends. But I was wrong. Her distress was linked to memories of severe physical pain because her shoes were so tight. She didn't tell her mum. Julie believed she couldn't bring additional burdens to an already heavily burdened mum. She feared that her needs would cause the family greater stress and that it could all fall apart. She therefore learnt to suffer in silence, not only as a child but most of her adult life. Her tears arose from a lifetime of unexpressed needs and fear of burdening anyone. Telling her story and putting the pieces together in therapy changed that. Without therapy, she likely would have suffered for the remainder of her life.

And that is why your story is vitally important, and why you, and only you, can make sense of it.

HOW DO I CONNECT MY PAST TO MY PRESENT?

Now that you have told your story, in this chapter I'll talk you through how to make sense of it. We're going to connect the past events of your life with who you are today. This will help you understand why you are the way you are.

Our first exercise is all about figuring out what you are struggling with in your life *now*.

Then we're going to look back through your timeline and figure out which event or period in your life might have been the cause of this struggle. The all-important *why*.

Finally, we can begin to look at possible solutions to the issues you're struggling with. These solutions will incorporate techniques that you'll later be employing in your daily practice.

Remember, we're just doing the foundation work here. We'll look at how you become your own therapist further on but for now, we're simply focusing on answering these questions:

- **What do you struggle with now?**
- **How might your story explain your issues?**

WHAT DO YOU STRUGGLE WITH NOW?

I realise this is a tricky question, and if you're anything like me the answer will change daily. And that's totally normal. Our thoughts, feelings and reactions to life are always in a constant state of flux, just like the weather. There will, however, be negative themes that recur again and again. It's just that our lives are so busy, we might not be conscious of the issues that routinely plague us until we choose to be actively aware of our moods, thoughts and behaviours. This is why we're going to be working on bringing your awareness to your fluctuating emotional states. Once you're equipped with an awareness of the main psychological challenges that are holding you back, you can choose to make changes in your life that will help resolve these issues. Awareness helps put you back in the driving seat of your life.

––––––––––

It's amazing how we can go from feeling like the Dalai Lama to the Hulk in a second.

I was recently taking a walk in the countryside, meditating and feeling at peace with the world. Ten minutes later I fell unceremoniously into a ditch and found myself covered in cow dung. It's fair to say that my thoughts and emotions changed quickly as I scrambled to my feet, dropping a few f-bombs along the way!

Thankfully, I was able to restore my sense of balance and laugh at the situation – something I've learnt through therapy. But many people struggle to manage their responses to the ups and downs of everyday life and get stuck in very unhelpful emotional states. If this sounds familiar, perhaps certain situations trigger negative emotional cycles in you.

You might be finding it hard to get to grips with what your main issues are. I have a bit of insight that might help. Having worked in healthcare for thirty years, I've witnessed a great deal of physical and psychological suffering first-hand, and in that time, I've noticed that most people's struggles fall into one of four main categories.

The research in most therapy disciplines will support my experience, but some models simply use different language.

The four key areas of struggle tend to be around:

1. **Lack of self-worth**
2. **Not feeling safe and secure**
3. **A sense of hopelessness**
4. **Questioning your lovability**

We'll go into more detail about each of these in a moment. Note how they are all linked to the third layer of the cake we spoke about earlier: your foundation core beliefs.

There are also natural 'personal struggle sub-themes'

that accompany each of these categories. For example, someone with low self-esteem might also feel socially anxious. So, that might mean that you're experiencing a cluster of different psychological struggles, all of which you initially believe you need to tackle separately, when in fact they are all related and can be approached effectively together.

Or it might mean that your main psychological obstacle doesn't seem to be explicitly covered by any of these categories, but it is in fact closely linked to one of them.

When it comes to the human condition, nothing is ever black and white. Whatever you struggle with, try to work out how it links to one of the four themes.

Recognition of what you may be struggling with is crucial. It's impossible to move forward without some degree of insight. And I discourage any of the following brush-offs that I hear daily:

- 'It's not that bad.'
- 'It could be worse.'
- 'Other people are worse off than me.'
- 'No point dwelling on that.'
- 'That's just the way I am.'

If you're smiling reading this list, then I'm probably talking to you!

Let's look at the four areas of struggle in more detail, and remember to keep in mind how your everyday struggles might link in with some or all of these.

THE FOUR AREAS OF STRUGGLE

1 LACK OF SELF-WORTH

Low self-worth can take many different forms and can lead to very different behaviours and feelings in different people. But fundamentally, low self-worth is a sense of either feeling 'less fundamentally valuable than other people', 'inadequate' or 'not good enough', despite there being no evidence to back up any of these negative feelings. It can manifest in many ways, ranging from a lack of confidence, avoiding people or situations, self-limiting beliefs, or battling with an inner dialogue that has strong tones of doubt, questioning, self-deprecation or even self-loathing. *It's living with a sense that you are lacking. It's living apologetically. It's living uncomfortably.*

Other people will appear better off than you and nothing you do will ever feel enough. Low self-worth will impact your home life, personal life, work life, and every aspect of your world. Everything might feel like it's an uphill battle. You may seek out ways to soothe this via alcohol, drugs, food or any substances that alter your state of mind. Alternatively, you may find yourself engaging in patterns of people-pleasing, overcompensating, perfectionism and opting out of life events that you don't feel worthy of.

Life can become all about trying to hide, or make up for, you 'not being good enough'. If this applies to you, particularly if you're only just realising it, this section may be a little hard to read, and you might even have some uneasy feelings stirring now. The discomfort is important and a healthy sign. Don't run away from it as it will bring you to the realisation that you are good enough, more than good enough.

2 NOT FEELING SAFE AND SECURE

Feeling safe and secure is noted as a priority in all therapy models. A feeling of safety and security is also important for our development. When we feel safe and secure, we tend to flourish in all aspects of life. On the other hand, when we feel unsafe or threatened, we struggle. In other words, we are anxious. Unfortunately, not everyone grows up in environments that feel safe and secure. Many homes are dominated by conflict. Many neighbourhoods are rife with crime. Many people feel threatened if they are in any way different, e.g. in terms of their skin colour, race, sexuality, religion or gender. I meet many people who grew up in countries with war, division and oppression. I also encounter a lot of people who have experienced violence, threats, abuse, bullying or humiliation, sometimes even from family members.

In summary, we live in a very imperfect, sometimes unsafe, messy, unpredictable world. Consequently, many people understandably enter adulthood feeling unsafe, vulnerable and frightened. Their brains have been hardwired to feel constantly threatened and anxious. The issue is exacerbated by the belief that they should be strong, resilient and in control, but they're failing. Therapy techniques can help to rewire the brain so it's less predisposed to feel under constant threat.

3 A SENSE OF HOPELESSNESS

Have you ever noticed that young babies smile at anyone? They don't judge. They don't see bad in people. They stare at everything with a sense of awe and excitement at all the possibilities. The world is a place to be explored. They are easily satisfied; all they need is food, drink, shelter and love. They cry when their needs are not met but they tend to settle when at ease (which is most of the time). I can imagine some parents rolling their eyes now, perhaps following a sleepless night!

But this is not a forever state. Babies soon grow up, absorbing every interaction, experience and situation. Depending on context and circumstance, some learn that the world is a safe place while others learn it's frightening and unsafe. When it comes to the latter, the people they encounter may be angry, dissatisfied, disillusioned or absent. The environments they encounter may be tough and sometimes impoverished. Money, food and employment may have been, or continue to be, scarce. The language surrounding them could have been negative and pessimistic. Hope is for other people, they are told, either explicitly or implicitly.

These experiences are their norm, so mood issues, depression and lack of motivation become the norm. The path to a niggling sense of hopelessness is set.

People don't choose to be hopeless. They become weary and worn out. Hopelessness is symptomatic of experiences. But thankfully new experiences can be created, and healing can occur. Hope is possible. I have witnessed this every day of my career over the last thirty years. Therapy is driven by hope, and you will experience it in our work together. If you're feeling a sense of hopelessness right now, I promise it *can* get better. It just takes a little time and effort.

4 QUESTIONING YOUR LOVABILITY

Have you ever noticed how many hit songs focus on love, heartache and loss? 'All you need is love.' 'Can't help falling in love.' 'I will always love you.' 'Can't buy me love.'

Love captures us. It sells products. We are told it makes the world a better place. Whatever your definition of love, there's no doubt most of us want it.

Love means feeling connected, seen, heard and understood by another human being. We crave a sense of belonging and to know we are not alone. In the absence of love we may wonder, 'Am I lovable?'

But we don't necessarily need to be single to question how lovable we are. Some people find themselves asking the same question when they're in a loving relationship, sometimes because of prior relationships or experiences. I heard a great expression from a Jesuit priest many years ago: 'If you really knew me, would you still love me?' What it means is that many of us doubt our lovability because we believe that our imperfections make us inherently less lovable. I believe our vulnerabilities make us more lovable.

If you've *never* been told that you're loved, then it's logical to doubt your lovability. But that doesn't make it true. Not everyone knows how to express love. I came from a family where there was love but the word itself wasn't used very often. This may be true for you too.

There is another possibility I would like you to consider. There are people in your life who may not have loved you in the way they should have. This doesn't mean you were not deserving of love, but it's possible that some of these people genuinely didn't know how to give it. For example, some people have a parent who doesn't know how to express love to them. They simply don't know how to do it. But we must also consider that love was never shown to them. Unexpressed love or an inability to express love can be transgenerational. An expression I come back to often that articulates this well is, 'Everyone is at fault, but no one is to blame.'

Whatever your experience has been of love, knowing you are lovable is pivotal to a full, happy life. To ignore that would be a travesty. Together, we will face your belief that you are not lovable (if indeed that is a belief you hold) head on, because whoever you are, whatever your story, whatever mistakes you've made, you are lovable. We all are. We are born that way.

OVER TO YOU FOR A LITTLE WORK

I can hear you sigh, but it will be worth it.

Let's break the work down into manageable chunks, exploring how you think, feel and behave, in relation to the four areas we've just covered. You may not need to cover all four areas; it could be that one area feels particularly pertinent to you. For example, if feeling safe and secure isn't a big issue for you, then it's fine not to dwell on that. You are in the driving seat here and it's your decision what you focus on.

I should preface this by saying that therapy isn't like a visit to a spa. You won't always feel pampered and indulged. There will be moments when you may not like what I say. You may feel like throwing the book at the wall or calling me some lovely swear words. Don't worry, I've heard them all before. I'm sure it must have been a therapist who came up with the well-worn phrase, 'No pain, no gain.'

But on the upside, therapy is transformative, and I guarantee you won't look back. I've said this before but it's worth reiterating now: many people can be disappointed when therapy doesn't feel 'good' all the time. But it shouldn't! Growth is hard work.

Uncomfortable moments can often be the most powerful. Sometimes when you connect with something that is truthful, it may feel difficult. You may feel a sense of resistance, anger, sadness, frustration, or want to avoid the feelings that are coming up. I strongly encourage you to stay with the feelings as much as possible. They are there for a reason and they serve a purpose – try to remember that when the self-therapy experience feels difficult. It will empower you.

EXERCISE 1

HOW TO RECOGNISE YOUR STRUGGLES

When you have decided which of the four areas of struggle you want to give your attention to, block out time to focus on *one at a time* somewhere quiet where you won't be interrupted. If possible, aim to spend thirty minutes on each. I suggest you work through the questions below for each of the areas of struggle, taking notes as you go. For example, if you are working through **hopelessness**, keep that theme in mind as you ask yourself the questions.

You may find that some of the questions touch

on similar areas and you're giving the same sort of answers. This is normal.

A reminder again of the four areas and everyday examples that may link to them:

- **Lack of self-worth:** feels like low confidence, self-doubt, fear of risk, self-criticism, not feeling deserving, not feeling good enough
- **Not feeling safe and secure:** feels like anxiety, can lead to panic attacks, phobias, avoidance of new situations, dislike of new routines, hyper-vigilance
- **A sense of hopelessness:** can mean depression, a lack of motivation, giving up on life, avoiding situations and people, lack of self-care, destructive behaviours
- **Questioning your lovability:** can result in relationship difficulties, not valuing yourself, accepting poor behaviour from others, negative appraisal of yourself, not prioritising your own needs, speaking negatively about yourself

A reminder that *this stage is simply acknowledging and recognising* what you may struggle with. Whatever comes up, just try to stay curious about how you react.

QUESTIONS TO REFLECT ON FOR EACH OF THE FOUR AREAS:

1. Do I have ways of thinking about myself, others and life that feel particularly negative, critical, fearful or catastrophic? Do I doubt myself and others, or am I cynical about others' intentions?

Make a note of whatever came up for you, as well as any other unwelcome or unhelpful ways of thinking not listed here and the situations during which those feelings surfaced. When does this happen for you? How often? Are there particular triggers or situations? It could be that reflecting on these questions makes you feel an unexpected emotion or leads to thoughts about something else. Remember you are simply noting what happens and not trying to work it all out at this stage. If specific examples come to mind, then of course, write them down. For instance, you may recognise you have a pattern of deflecting or refusing praise, a recent example being when you made a birthday meal for your partner yesterday but brushed off the compliments and said it was 'nothing', despite it taking you several hours to put together. There will be many examples that come to mind. Essentially you are bringing to life how your patterns play out in your everyday life.

NEXT, WE'RE GOING TO LOOK AT FEELINGS.

2. Do I regularly find myself feeling fearful, vulnerable, unsafe or lonely in my everyday life? Do I routinely feel sad, misunderstood, empty or isolated? Is a sense of abandonment the norm for me?

Make a note of whatever came up for you, as well as any other unwelcome or unhelpful ways of thinking not listed here and the situations during which those feelings surfaced. Reflect on any particularly pertinent examples from your everyday life that exemplify this issue. Ask yourself: are there some feelings that crop up more regularly than others? What do you do with these feelings when they arise? For example, do you try to block or stop them?

NEXT, WE'RE GOING TO LOOK AT YOUR
BEHAVIOURS. THIS IS WHERE IT GETS
REALLY INTERESTING.

3. Do I sometimes find myself behaving
   destructively? For instance, by drinking too
   much, taking recreational drugs, bursts of
   defensiveness, shouting or aggression,
   devoting a lot of my time to blaming others,
   engaging in bullying behaviour or lying?

Make a note of whatever came up for you, as well
as any other unwelcome or unhelpful behaviours
not listed here that you've noticed in yourself.

Now that you have reflected and identified the
thoughts, feelings and behaviours surrounding the
four areas of struggle, I want you to hold on to one
thought and keep it with you throughout your
reading of this book and beyond.

*Everyone, including you, was born good enough.
Any belief to the contrary is a falsehood that you
were taught by people or circumstances.*

Our job together is to help you unlearn anything
dysfunctional or unhealthy. And to do that I need
to help you understand *how life experiences that have
happened to you influence who you are today.*

HOW MIGHT YOUR STORY EXPLAIN YOUR ISSUES?

It's common for there to be more than one root cause behind our main areas of struggle. It's worth remembering that as children and in our formative years, our brains are like sponges, absorbing everything we hear and experience. Children can't differentiate using emotional intelligence the way an adult can. If someone calls a child 'stupid', 'fat', or 'ugly' regularly, then they may begin to normalise this as a truth. If, as a child, you are compared with a sibling and told they are brighter or better looking than you, then that sense of being 'of less value than other people' begins to kick in.

In my experience, much of the damage normally occurs at home. My intention here is not to blame parents or families, simply to offer the truth as I see it. Many families operate from dysfunctional foundations. They don't intend to cause harm, but they do. You know the script: 'Why can't you be more like your brother?', 'Stop whining and leave me alone' or 'You're lazy, selfish and ungrateful.'

Within many homes there are patterns of comparing, undermining, ignoring, criticising, judging or placing high expectations on a child, and this can cause problems. When this happens regularly, the negative message (whatever it is) is reinforced, which, in turn, influences the brain's neuropathways and our learnt emotional responses. I'll give you an example.

A child is told by his parents he is going to be a great football player when he grows up. His father wants him to play for England. They want a successful career for him, but the child has average skills at the game. Each time he comes home from a football game he is criticised by his father for not playing well enough, and told he should work harder. This happens after most games and the child feels humiliated and that he is a 'let down'. He then begins to develop a sense that he is of *less value* than other people and *not good enough*. A new neuropathway is consequently formed in his brain which conditions him to believe that unless he's successful, he's not good enough. His worth is compromised. Low self-worth is set in place.

These negative influences can also be found beyond the family home, within different cultures, religions, schools, gender stereotyping and of course all forms of media (social media especially). We are surrounded by people telling us who we should be, how we should be and what we should be! As a gay man, I am more than familiar with the detrimental impact these influences can have, and the importance of rewriting that script.

I'm going to be honest about how my own self esteem took a battering because of negative influences.

As a gay teenager growing up in a working-class area of Belfast, where there were clear ideas about how men should behave, I was always going to struggle. My version of masculinity didn't match up with that of the people around me and I didn't always fit in. I couldn't play football, for example, so I was at times ostracised. A question began to form in my mind, 'Am I not enough?' Culture and environment played a role in my feelings of low self-worth.

I grew up Catholic and listened to hundreds of sermons as a child telling me that *people like me* would go to hell. When I got older and became more conscious of my sexuality, I remembered those sermons and they made me wonder whether I was less worthy than other people. Later, I'd wonder, 'Am I a bad person?' Religion played a role in my feelings of low self-worth.

I went to a primary school that encouraged its pupils to excel in sports and praised sporting excellence above other skills and talents, but I far preferred music over sports. Again, more reinforced messages about not quite fitting in or being good enough.

I'm sure you get the picture. Various influences contributed to feelings of self-doubt and, over time, these became habitual. But my salvation was in finding a therapist and making sense of them. The circumstances I'd found myself in reinforced the lie that something was inherently wrong with me. But the truth was, I was completely fine. This insight changed everything for me.

I hope you can experience a similar revelation in your therapy with me.

HOW DO YOU LINK YOUR STORY TO WHAT YOU STRUGGLE WITH NOW?

So far, you've identified the biggest issues you struggle with, and you've told your story in full.

Now we're going to piece them both together (like the jigsaw I mentioned earlier). You want to be asking yourself the question:

What parts of my story can help me understand why I might sometimes have *low self-esteem, not feel safe or secure, experience feelings of hopelessness or not consider myself to be lovable?*

As before, if emotions or reactions come up as you're reflecting on or answering the questions, simply take note and allow them to be. Ideally you want to be curious about any emotional responses that crop up without being distracted by them.

EXERCISE 2

HOW TO CONNECT YOUR STORY TO YOUR EVERYDAY STRUGGLES

First, I invite you to go back and read over your story and see if anything immediately grabs your attention or helps you make a connection with what you struggle with today in relation to the four areas we have explored. For example, Jason, a client of mine, noticed a recurring theme in the subtle messages he'd received from his family throughout his life: avoid getting excited by life and you'll prevent disappointment. It was almost a family motto. As an adult he identified that this was one of the contributing factors to his intermittent episodes of depression and feelings of hopelessness.

You are looking for those 'Aha!' or 'lightbulb' moments. Moments when you think, 'My struggle finally makes sense.' Take note of any thoughts that emerge.

Here are some reflective questions that might help you out.

1. How might my family and home life have impacted upon each of my main areas of struggle today?

e.g. Was I valued, respected and listened to?

2. How might my community or environment have impacted upon each of my main areas of struggle today?

e.g. Did I fit in? Was I included?

3. How might my church or religion have impacted upon each of my main areas of struggle today?

e.g. Did this part of my life make me feel good?

4. How might my time at school or college have impacted upon each of my main areas of struggle today?

e.g. Was I bullied or humiliated?

5. How might any key incidents in my life have impacted upon how I see myself today?

e.g. Was I a carer for a family member? Was I over-weight or did I have acne as a teenager? Was I sexually assaulted?

6. How might my relationships (family, friends, work, romantic) have impacted upon each of my main areas of struggle today?
e.g. Can I recall any relationships that were destructive?

7. Detail anything else in your story that is significant for you in relation to the issues you struggle with and how you see yourself.

Here is a brief recap on where we are at this stage. Therapists love a recap, bear with me.

So far, you have:

- Told your life story in full without filter or self-judgement
- Identified your main areas of psychological struggle
- Connected your story with your struggles
- Gained a better understanding of why you might struggle

In the next chapter we're going to continue the foundation work by looking at what exactly you want to change in the future based on what you now know about yourself.

People make the mistake of thinking therapy is

all about talking. It's not! It is a way of life based on talking, feeling, responding, and knowing what you want and what you're doing. Think of it like training for a marathon: you need to do more than join the gym and buy new trainers. I'm going to be giving you the tools so that this way of living becomes second nature to you.

This work is about moving forward. I can't assume to know what you want for your future. But what I can say is: salvage what you can from your experiences and allow them to be part of a brighter future. We can't take a shortcut through the difficult parts, but the efforts you put in now will be paid back tenfold.

4

OK, WHAT NOW?

I'm sure you've heard of the expression 'to open Pandora's box'. According to Greek mythology, this box, once opened, was meant to release all the ills of the world onto mankind. It's an expression I often hear from people who are hesitant about engaging in therapy. 'I don't want to open Pandora's box. Who knows what will come out?' They're understandably concerned that therapy will dredge up painful memories long buried, and they're sceptical about it ultimately being a healing process. But this concern is unfounded.

The only thing you find when you explore your story is the truth. And as a wise person once said,

'The truth will set you free.' Even if you don't like the truth or the darker side of your story, it will ultimately lead you to a better life. When you find the courage to identify the formative experiences that have made you the person you are today, you will be empowered to reclaim ownership of your life and to discover what changes are needed. And that's what we'll be talking about in this chapter: daring to imagine a better future and changing your life.

But first, let's talk about the fear of change that can hold us back from that better future.

I'll often meet clients who aren't remotely wary of therapy. They'll tell me their story no problem, make sense of it, but then freeze. Suddenly they're faced with the reality that the future can be different from what they'd originally envisioned, and while for some people that can be liberating, for them it's terrifying!

Selena is a woman I welcomed into my therapy room a few years back. She had been diagnosed with a serious medical condition but thankfully had a very positive prognosis. She was at a crossroads in her life and described her serious illness as a 'wake-up call'. We got off to a great start in therapy. She was candid, honest, worked hard, didn't avoid issues and was open to suggestions. But this changed after a few sessions when I asked her, 'OK *what now?* What do you want for your future?' She couldn't speak and the atmosphere in the room turned cold. I was a little baffled. She had told me her story and got to the bottom of why she struggled in some areas of her life, but she wasn't able to go any further. My question had clearly upset her, and she decided there and then that therapy wasn't for her. She didn't want to continue, not today, not ever. I tried to explore this with her, but she was resistant.

As Selena was about to leave the room, I held the door open for her. I was a little taken aback by her keenness to exit, so, being unsure of what to say, I adopted a silent, calm demeanour (one of the tricks of the trade when you have a challenging moment as a therapist). I decided, as Selena was leaving, to keep the door open for some fresh air before my next client. But Selena automatically started to pull the door closed. I politely pulled it open again, gesturing my intention, but she pulled it back. To anyone watching in the waiting area I'm sure it looked like a tug of war between therapist and client. During this kerfuffle, I diplomatically and calmly informed Selena that I would like to leave the door open. She stopped and said, 'I'll think about it.' She thought I meant I wanted to keep the door open to future therapy with her!

I think back to this episode often as the perfect demonstration of both our unconscious wishes manifesting in our seemingly unrelated actions (on my side) and Selena's interpretation of those actions (on her side). While my conscious mind told me I was simply leaving the door open to get some fresh air, in fact I was keen for Selena to return to therapy and work through what she wanted for her future. And Selena's correct interpretation of my unconscious wish indicated her subconscious desire to return to therapy also. Significant meaning often lies beneath seemingly insignificant or unrelated actions. Psychoanalysts talk a lot about this, but we won't go into that here.

A week later Selena arranged to come back for a session. It's not uncommon for someone to drop out of therapy at difficult moments and then return after some thinking time. We explored what was going on for her. She had never worked out what she wanted for her life. No one had ever asked her what she wanted. She was a people pleaser. She avoided decision-making, and allowed other people to make decisions for her or for events outside of her control to 'carry her along'. My question forced her to face up to both this hard truth, and the prospect that she might have to abandon the patterns she'd established in her life that felt familiar and safe. I was asking her to look at a life full of new possibilities. And rather than inspiring excitement, this terrified her. Thankfully, she was able to identify that fear was getting in the way. We worked on that together successfully.

I wonder at this moment if you are experiencing a similar reaction to Selena when I ask the question, *What now? What do you want for your future?* Pause for a second and notice how it makes you feel.

Perhaps you can identify some of the following emotions:

- Vulnerability
- Reluctance
- Cynicism
- Doubt
- Fear
- Anxiety
- Instability
- Excitement
- Hope
- Curiosity
- Freedom
- Relief

There isn't a right or wrong answer here. There are no cash prizes. There are no booby prizes. If you had a negative reaction to the question about your future, that's completely fine. Your reaction could be telling you that fear, or old ways of thinking, are getting in the way of you envisaging a positive future for yourself. The good news is you can do something about that.

Likewise, a positive reaction could be a reminder that you are capable and ready to change.

The amazing benefit of therapy is that both positive and negative responses to questions about your future can be turned to your advantage. You could be feeling frightened, doubtful or vulnerable, but then turn these emotions into something powerful. As I've said before, therapy doesn't always feel good, at least initially. But together we can deal with all the emotions that come up. We can even thank them for supporting us (which is part of their function). Emotions work with us in helping us navigate our way through life. They are like an internal watchguard of sorts. Some of the emotions you'll experience during self-therapy may have felt overwhelming when you were a child, but as an adult you can now handle whatever comes up. Sometimes you just need to remind the child within you (and we all have one) that your adult self is on the case.

HOW HAPPY ARE YOU WITH YOUR LIFE RIGHT NOW?

Before you consider your future, it's important to review what's going well in your life and what isn't going so well.

We're going to do an exercise now that will encourage you to take a step back and assess how satisfied you are with the different areas of your life at this present time. The results of this exercise will act as a baseline that you can measure against in the future.

I want you to stop and consider how content you are right now with each life area that I've listed out below, then rate each out of 10 according to this scale.

8–10: Very satisfied
6–7: Reasonably satisfied
5: Could be a lot better
1–4: Dissatisfied

If there are any areas that I've left out but which are important to you, feel free to add them in.

- Achievements to date
- Work/school/professional life

- Finances
- Your home (by this I mean happiness with your home life, practically and emotionally)
- Where you live
- Social status
- How you look
- Friendships
- Romantic life
- Spirituality
- Family life
- Fun and adventure
- Self-confidence
- Values and principles
- Self-care (looking after yourself, physically, emotionally, psychologically)
- Physical health
- Mental health
- Hopes for the future
- Work/life (or study/life) balance
- Rest or relaxation time
- Making a difference to others or the world
- Looking after the planet
- General sense of satisfaction with all your life

How was that exercise for you? Some people find it enlightening. Let's face it, we rarely stop to evaluate our lives. We're all too busy working, looking after our families, scrolling Instagram or watching Netflix, to work out what we want.

Whatever your rating in each of the areas of your life, please don't be hard on yourself. If, for example, you arrived at a 4 or less in several categories, that's OK. It's better to be aware of your dissatisfaction than be in denial about it, as this helps you recognise which areas of your life might need a little work or more attention, and which have the biggest impact on your feelings of contentment. For instance, it may not be important to you that you have or make a lot of money, but so long as you feel like you're making a difference in the world, you're happy. Or you may identify that, so long as you're feeling connected to your partner and getting a daily workout in, you're generally content and can deal with anything life throws at you – whether that be a disappointment at work, or whether your finances or sleep or opportunities to have fun take a hit.

Equally, it's useful to acknowledge your areas of satisfaction.

It won't come as any great surprise to hear that almost every new client I meet is unhappy with their life. Not only that, but they can always list a few reasons (most of which are outside of themselves – we'll come to that) why they are unhappy. These reasons tend to be the direct result of dissatisfaction with the specific areas of their lives that they consider to have the biggest impact upon their feelings of contentment. So, either they've not recognised that these are the areas of their life that matter most to them, or they've not been working to keep their satisfaction levels in these areas 'topped up' (which it is their responsibility to do, as it is yours).

Here are some of the most common reasons clients cite for being unhappy with their lives. You might identify with one or more of these:

- My husband/wife/partner is a pain
- Life is too stressful
- I'm so busy all the time
- I've had a terrible life
- I hate my job/boss/work colleagues
- If I were richer, I'd be happier
- The kids are wearing me down
- I wish I'd made better choices
- It's all too much
- I can't get over what happened to me

So, we've acknowledged that our happiness is dependent on understanding which areas of our lives matter most to us. And we've acknowledged that *some* of these areas, such as where we live, or our past experiences with family or friends, or life-changing health issues or injuries to ourselves or others, fall outside of the realm of how we feel and behave, and of our identity today.

But it's equally important to be aware that these external factors are not *entirely* responsible for how we feel and behave.

Of course, some life events and current situations will have had a major effect on your feelings of contentment, and I don't want to minimise the impact they've had on your life, mental health and wellbeing (particularly if you've experienced deep loss, trauma or adversity).

But if we believe circumstances, many of which are outside of our control, are entirely responsible for who we are now, we can be left feeling powerless or like victims.

There is another option: we have choices in how we manage the harsh cards life may have dealt us. Once you realise that, you're empowered to act. Everything can change. 'I can't manage,' becomes, 'I have survived tougher moments.' 'This isn't fair,' becomes, 'What can this teach me?' 'My life is pointless,' becomes, 'My life has possibilities.' 'I will never get through this,' becomes, 'I am getting there.'

I appreciate this might be a little uncomfortable to read, but, for most people at least, it's the truth. We don't realise that we have a major part to play in our psychological wellbeing and happiness. Life happens to all of us, but how we react is everything.

You may have worked out by now that I want to guide you sensibly on to the *'What now?'* stage of our work. Your life satisfaction scores will help you consider what changes you would like to make for the future. For example, if you scored 3 on where you live, or your job, then of course it makes sense to look at ways of making changes in those areas. But I can't emphasise enough that your internal world need not take a back seat. Look at the scores relating to your mental health, self-care, hopes for the future, self-confidence, and values and principles. Consider how you think and deal with emotions. If your internal world isn't managed well, then you will continue to suffer. *If the inner world is neglected, the external world won't fill the void of dissatisfaction.*

WHAT DO *YOU* WANT IN THE FUTURE? WHAT DO *YOU* WANT TO CHANGE?

Now that you've looked back at your life story and used it to help you understand who you are today, and you've taken stock of how you feel about your life now, it's time to look forward. I'm going to ask again, what do *you* want your future to be? More of the same? Something better? A new start? Something extraordinary?

This is huge. You are at a crossroads, and you have the chance to take a different route with your life. Stop and ask yourself: are you prepared to settle for a humdrum life, or do you want to create something exceptional? The only person who can answer this is you.

I do want to share one thought as you ponder this. I spent ten years of my career in palliative care, watching people of all ages die, often unexpectedly and quickly. I am confident that most of those people, given a second chance, would have opted for more extraordinary moments in their lives. Whatever 'extraordinary' means for you, make your life count. And remember: 'extraordinary' doesn't mean bigger, better or more grandiose. It can be found when you decide to be fully present in the ordinary moments.

I've broken the question down into two essential components:

1. Tangible, material life changes you want for the future
2. The internal changes you want to make (ways of thinking, managing emotions, behaviours). Chapters 1 and 2 will help you

identify what changes you personally would benefit from making in this area

As with previous exercises, I am going to encourage you to take time out and consider the first of these questions carefully. You might have heard this stage described as 'goals', 'plans', 'targets' or 'aspirations' in other books. These are all great, but I would encourage you to think in terms of reclaiming life, hopes, contentment and peace. We're diving inward here.

I've noticed as a therapist that most people, when discussing future wishes, automatically direct attention to the external stuff: money, job, house, car, weight loss, relationships, etc. I get it. I'm as guilty as everyone else. No judgement here. I'd love more hair. I'd love a Porsche one day. I'd love to be as fit as I was when I was 20. I sometimes wish I had the looks of Tom Hardy. But somewhere deep down, I know it's not really me that wants that. My ego does, and that's OK. Our egos seek glory and gratification but if we know that and manage it, all is well. Ultimately egoic desire doesn't bring contentment. I know this personally. I see this with every client I work with. I'm sure it's the same for you. I've learnt from bearing witness to, talking about, and working to understand human suffering for more than thirty years, that material gains don't fully satisfy internal yearnings. Satisfaction and peace are primarily an inside job. I'm not saying here that you shouldn't have that holiday, buy that dress, change your eating habits. Go ahead and make the changes that are going to improve your life. I am, however, recommending that you also listen to the internal voice that whispers, 'Does this serve me well? Does this bring me peace?' The answer always comes.

I now hand over to you to make your list of what you want for your future, both material life changes and internal changes within yourself, keeping in mind the areas of life that matter most to you.

Did that exercise inspire you? I hope so.

I'd like us to work through one final task, keeping in mind what you want for your future. But before we get to that, I'd like to share Callum's story.

Callum is a recently qualified dentist I worked with recently who was struggling with anxiety and stress at work. He was a very engaged client and keen to change. When he completed his, 'What do you want for your future?' list, he agreed to read it to me at our session. It went something like, *I want to run my own practice by age 35. I want to drive a*

Range Rover. I want two children. As I listened, I was struck by the mechanical, dull tone of his voice. There didn't seem to be any passion for what he was saying. The way he spoke completely lacked energy. I commented on this, and he went quiet and looked at the ground for a long time before speaking. 'I've just realised, this is not my list. It's my father's.'

Callum's father was also a dentist and Callum had followed in his footsteps. His whole life, he'd felt immense pressure to please his father and live up to his expectations. Therapy was a very healthy choice for Callum. He was able to find his own voice and work out what *he* wanted for his life. He also had to work on making changes to unhelpful ways of thinking, some self-destructive behaviours, and to the direction of his career.

I invite you now to go back and read over your list of what you want for your future again, but this time, ask yourself these questions:

- Am I happy with this?
- Are these *my* needs and wishes (watch out for people-pleasing)?
- Will this bring me a sense of hope, peace and satisfaction?

Amend your list accordingly if you need to.

THE IMPORTANCE OF COMMITMENT AND PATIENCE

Two of the most common reasons people drop out of therapy, and the work involved, are difficulty committing and impatience. We are a generation focused on speed and convenience. We want everything instantly, including massive psychological and behavioural changes. If it isn't short, snappy and to the point, it's difficult to engage people.

Therapy, however, *does* require commitment and patience, and I'll explain why it's worth investing in both.

1. Commitment

I want you to think of your daily commitment to self-therapy as something you do for yourself, rather than as an onerous piece of work that must be slogged through. This is your opportunity to turn up for your life, maybe for the first time. Every time you engage with this work you are respecting yourself. Of course, there are also practical considerations. You are working on changing emotional patterns, and patterns of thought and reaction that will have been part of your life for a very long time. As you're essentially re-wiring your brain, this will require consistency, but the result will be an incredible ability to manage life completely differently.

A helpful way of thinking about this commitment is to have a key word you remind yourself of every time you're going off track. My key word is *sabotage*. I know it sounds strong, but that's a conscious decision. If I don't commit to looking after myself, then I am sabotaging my wellbeing. Something about saying that word serves the useful purpose of giving me a kick up the backside. Whatever word you decide on, use it when you need to and make sure it's a shocker! Use a word you will remember. It could be a cartoon character, something from a movie or anything that is relevant. What is crucial is that it acts as a clear signal to you that you are going off track.

A wise supervisor during my training reminded me that therapy without commitment is like using sunscreen made of cooking oil. It's totally ineffective and can make things worse. And he was right. There is no value in discovering who you are and how you function unless you are willing to do something about it.

This is a commitment for life. A better life.

2. Patience

I'm always amused when some clients, after a few sessions, tell me they're worried therapy isn't working. When I ask them what they'd hoped would happen, they tend to say that they would have liked for it all to have been sorted out (their life, that is). No pressure whatsoever after three sessions. It always makes me smile when this happens. I have a standard response every time: *'You will never have it all sorted out, even if you live to 100.'* And that's the truth. There is no blissful end state where all your troubles will have vanished, and you live happily ever after. That doesn't happen. Life, with all its up and downs, will continue to happen to you. It's how you respond to the ups and downs that's the key. Patience with the process will help enormously with how you manage life.

Let's talk about that word, 'process'. Therapy is often described as a process, and the very word implies patience. When I go to an art gallery, I am always struck by the detail that goes in to some of the great works. It reminds me of the hundreds of hours that will have been dedicated to the process. There will have been mistakes, sleepless nights, the ripping up and starting again, tears, disillusionment, and of course the age-old question, *Will this be good enough?* At the time, the painter won't know that it'll eventually become more than good enough. That it will become a masterpiece in the fullness of time. It is the painter's patience with the process that helps their painting attain greatness. The painter's talent becomes secondary to their patience.

What I encourage wholeheartedly is that you engage patiently. I think I've made my point about the importance of carving out time in your day to do the therapy itself. But more fortitude may be required when it comes to awaiting change to take place within you. You may find yourself falling into the following thinking traps:

- **Defeatist:** 'What's the point of this?'
- **Frustrated:** 'I don't have time for this.'
- **Impatient:** 'Why am I not feeling better?'
- **Avoidant:** 'This is not for me.'
- **Defensive:** 'This is all bull*hit.'
- **Denial:** 'I'm completely fine.'
- **Repression:** 'I'll do this another time.'
- **Persecutory:** 'I'm beyond help.'

As with the key word you're going to be employing when your commitment starts to falter, I encourage you to do the same when you sense your own impatience. If helpful, my phrase is '*missed opportunity*'. When I'm impatient I run the risk of missing something incredible.

We are all works in progress. Sometimes we need to be reminded not to place unrealistic expectations on ourselves and make things more challenging than they ought to be. Commitment and patience in therapy are both essential.

Speaking of the essential ingredients for effective therapy, the next chapter brings us on to the other therapy non-negotiables: tools, techniques and tips, employed alongside self-care and self-respect.

CHAPTER 5

ACTIONS SPEAK LOUDER THAN WORDS

By now, you'll have more insight into who you are and how you operate. You'll also have arrived at a vision of how you'd like to function psychologically, and feel, in the future.

We now move on to the doing: the *actions* of therapy. These are the therapeutic tools and techniques you can use during your daily self-therapy to tackle your personal psychological 'problem areas' that we identified in Chapter 3. They will change the way you think now to the way you want to think in the future.

We'll be revisiting the techniques you'll be learning

in this chapter in Chapters 6, 7, and 8, when I take you through your ten-minute self-therapy practice.

Therapy is often referred to as a 'talking therapy', but I find this to be a restrictive definition. Good therapy involves so much more than just talking. Talking is like stretching at the gym; transformation can only happen with actions.

Whatever you are struggling with, whether it be relationships, addiction, anxiety, depression, loss or any of the issues that make us human, action is a crucial part of the process. Talking gets the ball rolling, action brings about change.

In my experience there are four key **actions** and four **self-commitments** that need to be part of everyone's therapy, regardless of the issue. The actions and self-commitments go hand in hand.

THE FOUR ACTIONS OF THERAPY ARE:

1. **Restructuring how you think**
2. **Rewriting your rules and beliefs**
3. **Engaging in healthier behaviours**
4. **Engaging with life**

1. Restructuring how you think

As we know, thoughts can sometimes be problematic. Occasionally, they are hard to switch off. They can be negative, critical, burdensome, harsh, sabotaging, catastrophic, judgemental, unhelpful and fearful. On the other hand, they can also be helpful, rational, kind and a force for good. But the harsh reality is, negative thoughts tend to draw us in more. They have a magnetic quality. We are more likely to listen to negative thought patterns.

The problem is that we assume we have no control over our thoughts. That they're a fact of life that we need to put up with. And to an extent this is true.

But we also know, from our work earlier, that we can be programmed to think in certain ways in particular situations. And while that can be a problem, particularly if the thought patterns we've been programmed with are negative, this also means that we can program ourselves to have positive thoughts in certain situations, too.

We also tend to accept our thoughts as factual and truthful. This creates challenges because often they're not. Sometimes they are random and make no sense.

Finally, there is the issue of how we relate to our thoughts. For example, if you have a thought you deem 'bad', that doesn't mean you are a 'bad' person. It signifies you are human. There have been interesting studies with OCD research showing how random, nonsensical and out-of-character thoughts can sometimes be. We all have the capacity to have violent, sexual, angry or blasphemous thoughts that run counter to our values or belief systems. None of these thoughts define who you are but if you relate to them as if they do, then you will feel distress.

Just to be clear, I am not saying that all thoughts are to be ignored. Sometimes thoughts follow a rational process and are an important part of psychological processing, decision-making and staying safe. The key is to be able to identify the difference between a helpful, adaptive thought and an unhelpful, maladaptive thought. You might be wondering how to tell the difference. It's quite simple.

Unhelpful thinking patterns, although familiar, tend to contribute to distress and a sense of discomfort. They tend to be spontaneous, fast, repetitive and have a burdensome quality. Think of the last time you had some thoughts that were difficult to listen to: 'You're a failure,' 'This is going to go wrong,' 'Don't speak, people will laugh at you,' for example. Such thoughts will alter your mood and increase your anxiety. They will feel uncomfortable.

On the other hand, helpful thinking presents differently. For example, you may have a decision to make or a task to complete. As you begin to think through the pros and cons of your decision, or the actions required to complete the task, your thoughts will feel appropriate and necessary. They are in context, whereas the former are fear-driven or misguided. It is worth mentioning here that anxious thinking isn't wrong. Some degree of anxiety can be healthy. But when the threat is exaggerated and not in context with the reality of the situation, it becomes problematic.

Back to how we can reprogram our negative thought patterns. There is a simple process for doing this and it involves four steps:

- Recognising an unhelpful thought pattern
- Examining the evidence to support the thought you're having. Is there irrefutable proof that what you're thinking is true? For example, you might consider applying for a job, then immediately think, 'I'll never get it.' Where is the evidence to support that as true?
- Replacing the thought with a more helpful alternative
- Letting go of the unhelpful thought

The incredible power of this technique is that each time you do it to disrupt unhelpful ways of thinking, you're encouraging your brain to respond differently in the future.

Up until now, you've never questioned the validity

of your thoughts, so your brain has continued to deliver these unhelpful thoughts on the basis that they're protecting you, by stopping you from doing things your brain believes are harmful. But when you start challenging them, your brain recognises that you're not buying into familiar thought patterns, and instead you've presented more rational, adaptive alternatives. You're starting to reprogram your mind to think more flexibly. From thereon in, your brain will start responding with healthier thoughts. You're literally getting one step closer to re-wiring your brain permanently each time you use this technique. This also means that each time you employ it will be slightly easier than the last.

Isn't that powerful? You don't have to be a victim of your thoughts. You are not your thoughts. You are free of the tyranny of your mind.

2. Rewriting your rules and beliefs

As you know from telling your story and linking it to your life, the unwritten rules and beliefs you live your life by are highly influential. They are your compass. You learnt as a child that if you behaved in a particular way it got you noticed, accepted, loved, respected and so on. You also learnt how to stay safe and minimise the risk of harm. These learnings became your rules and beliefs. The problem is these rules have probably never been reviewed in your adult life. They may not serve you well anymore.

I think of rules and beliefs as like wearing your favourite outfit. We all have clothes that can boost our confidence, stability and sense of ease. When I'm giving a talk, I always wear clothes that I like. If I wear a shirt that's a little tight (a regular problem since turning 40) or new shoes I haven't worn in, then I don't deliver as well. I'm showing up restricted, and it shows.

It's similar with rules and beliefs. If you are living according to rules and beliefs that don't work for you, it's restrictive and uncomfortable. It's like living in a straitjacket.

Rules and beliefs are usually prefaced with *must* and *should*. This is normally followed up with another belief about consequences. For example, *I must never lie. If I lie, something bad could happen to me* (common belief when religion is involved). I've mentioned this before but it's worth saying again: there is nothing wrong with rules and beliefs in themselves. When used well, they can support you and help with a sense of wellbeing and balance. It's when you start to believe there is no flexibility or choice with your rules and beliefs that the problems arise.

Patrick's story highlights this well. I met him a

few months after he had finished university. He graduated with a 2:1 and became depressed several weeks after his results were issued. Patrick was a straight-A student from childhood. He'd been president of the student union at university and was predicted a first-class degree.

When he didn't achieve his first, Patrick believed that he had not only failed himself but also his family. At one stage, he considered taking his own life. As we set out on Patrick's path to recovery, I discovered he held extremely rigid personal rules and beliefs. His 'shoulds' and 'musts' focused on never failing, never disappointing people, never saying no, always being the best. He was a perfectionist in every aspect of his life. Not achieving the degree he'd expected was his first experience of disappointment. His inflexible rules and beliefs didn't support him through this.

We worked on creating more flexibility and openness with his rules and beliefs, and slowly his depression began to lift.

'I must be the best,' was replaced with, 'I can only try my best.' 'I must not disappoint,' was replaced with, 'Sometimes I might disappoint, and that's OK.' 'I should always please people,' was replaced with, 'It's not always possible to please everyone.'

Patrick created flexibility with his rules and beliefs, and in turn his mood improved, he found freedom and openness, and became a much happier, more peaceful person.

The same process is also possible for you. I encourage you to make a list of all the 'shoulds' and 'musts' you've created for your life and ask yourself whether they can be made more flexible.

As you'll have realised by now, though, it's not just about making a list. We also need to work on putting your more flexible approach into practice. The next time you realise you're functioning from a place that's inflexible, stop. Acknowledge that you have the choice to review your rules and beliefs. You can opt for more flexibility.

3. Engaging in healthier behaviours

When we are having a difficult time, most of us seek out comfort in some way. You may notice that the extra drink in the evening, drugs, spending, distractions, sex or whatever works to soothe you, suddenly becomes habitual. Before going any further here, I want to assure you that the fun police haven't arrived! We all need some fun, lightness and distractions at times. But when behaviours come with negative consequences or get in the way of your life, it's time to reassess.

It's normal to want to numb your emotions, or distract yourself, or seek out escapism or endorphin rushes when life is challenging. But it's always a temporary solution. At some point you must return and face the music – that is, your day-to-day life.

Here, I'd like to encourage you to do some soul-searching and evaluate the behaviours in your life that could potentially be creating issues for you, the unhealthy ways that you're seeking comfort.

In my clinical practice, the problematic behaviours that I see tend to be centred around:

- Alcohol
- Drugs
- Food
- Sex
- Overspending
- Gambling
- Unhealthy relationships
- Conflict and anger
- Self-sabotaging
- Sleep
- Self-neglect
- Avoidance (not doing what you need to do)
- Delaying gratification (putting off things you enjoy)
- Defensiveness (feeling the need to protect and defend yourself)
- Anger (potentially overreacting to situations)
- Criticising (overly critical of others and yourself)

- Judging (making harsh judgements about others and yourself)
- Projecting (mistakenly believing others to feel what it is you feel but do not acknowledge)
- Withdrawing (socially pulling back, leading to isolation)
- Regressing (responding with more juvenile, childlike responses)
- Psychological inflexibility (not seeing other people's point of view)
- Being defeatist (giving up easily)
- Being in denial (not acknowledging what's happening)
- Self-focusing (not paying attention to the needs of others)

If these, or any other behaviours you can think of, are getting in the way of your life, I encourage you to think of ways of reducing, improving or stopping them. Sometimes this will require support. It may also involve substituting some of your behaviours with healthier alternatives. Again, I don't want to be prescriptive about this. I suspect you will intuitively know what you need to do. Most people do. A reminder again that a list of support organisations is provided at the end of the book.

I know this work isn't easy. I've said a few times

now that behaviours, choices and actions are important. A person can have all the insight in the world but unless they are willing to act, the work is pointless.

4. Engaging with life

In my career, I've been lucky enough to work alongside some exceptional people. People who care. People with incredible skills and empathy. As therapists we all have supervisors who are also therapists. Every therapist talks to another therapist to get support. It's like a daisy chain of support.

In one of my NHS jobs, I was supervised by a very intelligent and skilled psychiatrist. He was diagnostically sharp. I learnt a lot from him about psychiatric disorders, the importance of assessment and the role of medication with some people. He was also brutally honest, which I really liked.

I remember a discussion with him about a patient, Philomena, who was struggling with severe anxiety and depression. I had tried every technique and I was getting nowhere. I was feeling defeated and a little lost (my perfectionist rules and beliefs were winning out over adaptive thinking). My supervisor looked at me, and asked, 'Have you tried "life" with this patient?' Initially I was baffled. He went on to say, 'The antidote to pain is life.'

I asked him to elaborate, and he replied, 'Is your

patient engaging with any aspect of life: work, socialising, exercise, volunteering, a walk, a hobby, gardening?' And there – a sudden lightbulb moment. Philomena was naturally disengaging from most of her life, but she loved gardening. I, short-sightedly, hadn't considered it could be part of treatment.

My supervisor suggested I ease up on all the techniques and encourage Philomena to connect with her gardening. And that's exactly what I did.

As luck would have it, my job at the time was close to a gardening centre, and they were seeking volunteers! Fast-forward four weeks, following a lot of persuasion and patience: Philomena started her training there. Everything changed. She came alive in our sessions. Within weeks her symptoms improved. She became motivated. Her eyes sparkled. There was a lilt in her voice I'd never heard before. She had found the antidote to pain: gardening.

This experience changed how I work as a therapist. Of course, we need to follow a process and use therapeutic techniques, but we must include 'life' in the treatment plan, whether it be through a gym, a book club, Zumba, bird-watching, fishing or something else completely. All of life offers healing if we can find something to connect to.

And now I put this question to you: how engaged are you with life?

Stay with this question. Take time with it. Don't rush.

If you're going through a tough time right now, that's OK. Is there one part of life you could connect with a little more? It might feel difficult and you may need to start slowly. But that's fine. If you like walking, go for a five-minute walk today. It's a start. If you like nature, just go look at a tree today. It's a start. If you can do more, great. Do what you can.

When you connect with what interests or matters to you, your body releases the feelgood hormones serotonin, oxytocin and dopamine. You start to feel more connected to other people. Your motivation improves. Negative patterns crop up less and less frequently. You begin to heal.

Today I challenge you to take one step towards re-engaging with your life, particularly if you have been avoiding it. *The antidote to pain is life* has become something of a mantra for me. I think about it often. Maybe it can perform the same function for you.

The solutions you are seeking are likely to be closer than you think.

THE FOUR COMMITMENTS TO SELF

We now move on to look at what I call *the four commitments to self*. These are more of an internal job, a change of perspective if you like. You may be surprised at how deceptively simple, yet empowering, they are. They involve a shake-up of your approach to yourself. The four commitments are:

1. **Talking to yourself as though you're someone who matters (because you *do* matter)**
2. **Looking after yourself**
3. **Going easy on yourself**
4. **Showing up in your life authentically**

On average, most people, if they were rated for how well they performed in each of these areas, would get a very low score. I meet people from every walk of life in my line of work. The one common factor I see every day: *people don't treat themselves well.* I believe this is unquestionably the crux of the human struggle.

The most consistent part of your life is you. You will have you with you until your last breath. How you speak to yourself, how you treat yourself, how you look after yourself are symbols for your life. Whatever life throws at you, if you are in 'good company' with yourself, then the journey will be so much more manageable and enjoyable.

I went travelling to the US in my twenties – a cliché, I know! Partway through my trip, I met a fellow backpacker and we agreed to travel together for a month. But after one week, I was exhausted. He was negative. He complained about everything. He was critical. He was unappreciative. He was also very rude to most people he interacted with.

I tried hard to be compassionate, but I realised I couldn't travel for a full month with him. After the first week I told him I was going to travel alone and that's what I did. Even though I was anxious about solo travelling, I realised I could rely on the part of me that was kind, curious, open to adventure and generally keen to have a good time. I could be alone with myself.

In life, we need to learn how to become solo travellers because sometimes we might unexpectedly be alone, or circumstances might change. We need to learn the skill of being able to talk to ourselves in a positive tone. We need to learn how to look after ourselves. We need to learn how to be compas-sionate to ourselves. We need to be able to show up in the world, comfortable in our own skin. When we live this way, we adjust better to life's uncer-tainties and unpredictability. It's like living life in the presence of a reliable best friend. And that best friend is you.

1. Talking to yourself as though you're someone who matters (because you *do* matter)

We all have a running internal dialogue. Take a minute to stop and notice the chatter. It tends to sound something like this: 'Why did he say that?', 'Does my boss like me?', 'Is my partner bored with me?', 'I'm too fat,' 'I wish I was a better mum/dad.' And on and on it goes.

Our internal tone towards ourselves can often be destructive, harmful, judgemental, even cruel.

Clients often describe negative events in their life to me – events like conflict, hardship, loss or heartache. As they're describing these events, I always ask one question: *How are you talking to yourself in this moment?*

These are the type of responses I hear almost every time:

- I'm such an idiot
- I'm stupid
- This is my fault
- I'm pathetic
- I'm a waste of space
- I'm useless
- I'm a fool
- I'm a [insert endless list of expletives]

People talk to themselves like they don't matter. And that's exactly how that kind of internal chatter leaves them feeling. Our emotional response correlates with the tone and language we use towards ourselves.

If this is striking a chord with you, I have one suggestion: *Work on paying attention to the tone of your internal chatter. As soon as you feel it turning negative, shut that voice down. Calmly and firmly tell it to stop. You deserve better.* Once you've accepted that you matter, then you owe it to yourself to talk to yourself like you do. Change your tone. Change your language. Talk to yourself the way you would talk to someone you respect. The transformation will be instantaneous.

2. Looking after yourself

It might sound a little odd that I'm including this as part of therapy, but it's crucial. Self-care isn't high on the agenda for most people. I often deliver talks on mental health to large organisations. These I'll start by asking how many people have devoted time to self-care that day. On average I'm lucky if a dozen people raise their hand, and that can be in a room of 500 people!

Before we continue, let's first define self-care. Self-care is the act of looking after yourself physically, psychologically, emotionally or even spiritually. It doesn't necessarily mean taking a bath or having a massage (although it can mean both or either of these things, if that's what you really need). Eating a healthy diet, exercising, resting, mindfulness or meditation, seeing friends and family, and practising gratitude are all forms of self-care.

I encourage you to think of self-care broadly and evaluate truthfully how you look after yourself every day. Here are some questions to ponder:

- Does your diet support a healthy lifestyle?
- Do you manage to include some physical exercise (within your capabilities) into your day?
- Do you create breaks within your day?
- Do you engage in anything that helps quieten your mind?
- Do you talk about issues that are bothering you?
- How often are you connecting socially with others?
- Do you feel there is balance between your work and your non-working life?
- Do you prioritise other people's needs before your own?
- Do you express appreciation for the positives in your day?

Self-care can sometimes be misunderstood or portrayed as selfish, a luxury, or unrealistic considering the demands of modern life. I would challenge this. Self-care is *essential* for healthy daily functioning. It's responsible. It not only helps you get the best from *your* life, but others also experience the best of *you*. It is a powerful statement that you value and respect yourself. You are taking responsibility and ownership for your life. Earlier we discussed the impact of how you talk to yourself on how you feel about yourself. Self-care (or the lack of it) has a similar effect. Self-care is a therapeutic act. You are showing up in your life and deciding that you deserve looking after. Without self-care, the risk of exhaustion, burnout, breakdown – call it what you like – increases significantly. There is nothing fluffy or self-indulgent about self-care. It needs to be taken seriously. I see the darker side of people ignoring the warnings from their body that they need to take care of themselves. You have the choice to proactively change this today.

3. Going easy on yourself

I noticed a few years back that when I asked clients about self-compassion, they often threw me a suspicious glance. It could translate to, 'What snowflake wizardry is this man talking about?' That's when I started phrasing the question differently: 'Do you give yourself a hard time?' To *that* question I'd almost always get a resounding '*Yes.*'

I started following that question up with another: 'Do you think life would be easier if you did less of that?' Again, invariably a resounding '*Yes.*' This is the point at which I now suggest we talk about self-compassion.

Self-compassion is broader than how you talk to yourself. It's a much deeper level of self-care that is both mindset- *and* action-based. It means employing self-acceptance and warmth, it means dialling down the judgement and learning to comfort yourself in darker times.

It means saying, 'It's OK,' 'We can do this' and 'I'm with you' to yourself when it seems impossible. It means asking yourself the question, 'What do you need?' Self-compassion means you instinctively learn when to leap into action and when to stop, when to advocate for yourself and when to protect yourself, e.g. 'Let's take a break,' 'I'm taking you away for a holiday,' 'I want you to see less of these people' or 'Let's go out for a walk and switch off for a while.'

If I were forced to choose just one tool as a therapist, it would be self-compassion. Let me explain why. As humans we make mistakes. We screw up sometimes, we fail, we fall, we experience exhaustion and we are imperfect. And we persecute ourselves for all of that.

Self-compassion is powerful because it means accepting and sitting in our flawed humanity. Because this is very difficult for most people, practising self-compassion tends to cut right to the source of our issues. You learn to get to know the enemies within yourself and approach them with greater understanding, lightness and openness.

Self-compassion means embracing life as it is, and yourself as you are, now. It's not conditional on successes, achievements or accolades. If you are someone who gives yourself a hard time, try a self-compassionate approach. It is a loyal, faithful companion that you can access at any time, and it won't let you down.

4. Showing up in your life authentically

In a society that's obsessed with creating the illusion of perfect lives, perfect bodies, perfect relationships, perfect teeth and so on, I propose a different route. Simply show up unapologetically as you are.

I wholeheartedly believe that when we try to create an illusion that is at odds with who we are, we weaken our position. People sense inauthenticity immediately. We can feel it when we are around people who aren't sincere or genuine. If an authentic approach doesn't get you what you want, perhaps you are on the wrong path. If you dilute, minimise, or fabricate who you are, you compromise your integrity and the foundations supporting you.

I remember once being advised by a friend not to talk too much about my own struggles in book interviews because 'People don't want advice from a therapist who has struggled.' I disagreed and chose not to adapt my approach. I am good at my job partly because I personally have known, and I understand, human struggle. Why would I hide that? The best professionals in health and psychology are often those people who have walked the walk.

I'm not advocating that you shouldn't strive for self-improvement. Personal growth can fulfil you and help to augment those aspects of your personality and identity that make you special and unique. All I ask is that you avoid the trap of believing you need to be different from what you are. You don't.

Commit to your authentic self. It won't let you down.

PART 2

CHAPTER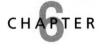

GET *READY* FOR
YOUR DAY

Have you ever had one of those days where you've rushed out of the house already late for an appointment looking like you've been dragged through a hedge backwards, with your jumper on inside out and just blindly hoping you've got your phone, wallet and keys with you? Apart from looking like you've just been on a motorbike without a helmet, you also notice that your mind is racing. Everything feels frantic, chaotic and imbalanced. You're not set up for the day and consequently the remainder of the day landslides into what can best be described as a pile of crap. We all have them.

Next time you're on a morning train or bus, or in traffic, observe how frazzled everyone looks. But it doesn't have to be this way.

Now you've completed the foundation work, we're going to incorporate your learnings into your everyday life.

One of most common misconceptions that exists around therapy is that it's a once-a-week chat, and that's it. Job done. But therapy is a way of life, and it needs to be so because life throws new challenges at you all the time. Once you've mastered the skill of navigating your way along life's twists and turns, you'll feel truly empowered.

Your ten minutes of daily self-therapy is a mix of proactive and reactive techniques that will help restore a sense of balance.

This chapter will focus on the first *four minutes of your daily ten-minute practice*. These four minutes get you **ready** for the day ahead the right way.

I must admit, I wasn't always a morning person. I wasted a lot of time faffing about, not achieving much. Therapy taught me to change that. How we start the day strongly influences how we experience the rest of it. Some of the research around mindfulness supports this.

I imagine many of you will be thinking about the volume of responsibilities you have each morning:

getting the kids up, doing the school run, walking the dog, making packed lunches, getting to work and so on. Now I'm adding another chore to your list! I accept that. But these four minutes will, I promise, change every aspect of your day. If you can spend a few minutes brushing your teeth and having a shower, then I strongly encourage you to find a few minutes to take care of your mind. It might even involve letting go of something else that isn't a priority.

HOW DOES THIS WORK?

Everyone's morning routine is different so I won't be prescriptive about exactly when in the morning this should be done. I simply ask that you fit these four consecutive minutes into the first few hours of your day. The earlier, the better. I just have one condition: that you find somewhere quiet and private for these four minutes to allow yourself space. If that involves locking yourself in the bathroom, then so be it. If noise is an issue, use headphones or ear plugs. Practically, I encourage you to find ways to make it work and be aware of the negative script that may pop up saying that it's 'impossible', 'I can't do this' or 'I don't have time.' Notice this voice and gently shut it down.

During these four minutes of self-therapy, we'll cover off four focus areas. I'm going to give you all the background, the context and the 'why' of your daily self-therapy practice as well as the 'how' over the following few pages, so the content covering your practice will look like a lot to take in at the first read-through. But don't worry. Only some of this relates to the 'how': what, practically, you'll actually be doing every day as part of your self-therapy.

Also, don't fret if you run over time to start with. This process will get easier as you become more familiar with it. Think of it like essential daily checks.

I want to reiterate that while the daily self-therapy I'm teaching you in this book is not a substitute for a full course of in-person therapy, putting aside these four minutes to kickstart your day is a hell of a lot better than taking no minutes. Most people dedicate zero time to therapeutic self-care. You are a step ahead of the game.

The four areas of focus are:

MINUTE 1 | Emotional regulation check-in: *How am I doing today?*

MINUTE 2 | A self-care strategy taken from compassion-focused therapies: *What do I need today?*

MINUTE 3 | A tool used in integrative therapy: *Gratitude and intention*

MINUTE 4 | A technique used in mindfulness and EMDR therapy (explained on p156): *Grounding*

MINUTE 1: HOW AM I DOING TODAY?

This involves tuning in to where you're at emotionally, physically and psychologically by curiously exploring each of the following questions:

- *How am I emotionally today?* What emotions are present and dominant? Here, we want to acknowledge your emotions and let them guide you in a way that will benefit you
- *How does my body feel?* Scan for any tension, discomfort and pain
- *What's my mind doing?* Observe the volume, speed and quality of your thoughts

I'll take you through how to perform each of these check-ins in a moment, but first, let's remind ourselves of why it's important to know how we're doing every day.

If we don't know how we are, then we won't know what we need. If we don't know what we need, then we won't look after ourselves properly. And that's a form of self-neglect, which leads to unnecessary suffering.

If you're a fan of the sitcom *Friends*, you will be familiar with Joey's infamous chat-up line, 'How *you* doin'?' It never ceases to make me laugh. It also pops into my head sometimes when I'm asking a client how they are. Naturally, I avoid asking, the question in Joey's signature flirty style (that would be disconcerting for clients!), but I try to avoid asking, 'How are you feeling?', which sounds clichéd to my ears. Additionally, at the start of therapy, it's sometimes hard to access and name your feelings, or you might not be ready to experience the vulnerability that shows up when you attempt to dive straight in and interrogate your feelings with a capital F. A more down-to-earth, open question tends to produce more useful replies that we can work with. This is why I suggest you start with 'How am I doing?' not 'How am I feeling?'

The reality is most people never take a moment to stop and check in with how they are. Most of the population wake up, roll out of bed and auto-pilot into the day. Let me put this another way. If we think of ourselves as a functioning body with the brain our main engine, why wouldn't we carry out daily maintenance checks? I'm sure most of us wouldn't fly with an airline that didn't check the engines before take-off. Why then don't we do the same before we take off into our day? It's a no-brainer!

HOW AM I EMOTIONALLY TODAY?

Assuming you are somewhere quiet, away from distractions, I suggest you start by sitting comfortably, feet apart and placed firmly on the ground. Close your eyes and place your hand on your heart or tummy area. The act of placing your hands on the parts of your body associated with emotion can help you become more aware of your emotional responses.

Next, gently ask yourself, *'How am I doing today, emotionally? What's going on?'*

If emotions such as a sadness or anger are present, they will emerge, and finding ways to express that will come. Asking the question with curiosity, openness, and compassion allows the emotion to reveal itself.

Remember, at this stage you are not trying to remove the emotion or do anything with it. You simply need to acknowledge it's there as this will inform how you plan your care for the day.

In the second minute of self-therapy, we'll consider what actions you'd like to incorporate into your day that will help soothe any negative emotions you find. For example, if you discover sadness, then self-care, an adjustment to your routine and speaking to a close friend could all be scheduled in to your day. This way, you're facing your emotions and saying to that part of yourself, *I hear you. I see you. I am here for you*. For now, though, you are simply self-soothing.

HOW DOES MY BODY FEEL?

There's an expression, *The body keeps the score*. What this means is that when we endure heartache, loss, trauma or adversity, the pain from these experiences is often held in the body. Our body remembers them. Sometimes a life event can activate these memories physiologically, and they manifest as bodily pain and tension. Just like emotions, that pain can serve as a barometer for how we're doing, even if consciously we've not acknowledged the depth of our distress.

Think about when you hear people say, 'I have a lump in my throat,' or 'My chest is pounding' or 'I feel like my head's going to explode,' but there seems to be no logical explanation as to why. Nothing's upset them that they're aware of, they haven't just run for the bus, they aren't frightened.

In these instances, it's possible they've triggered a negative memory, and they're experiencing that memory physically rather than psychologically. It's a reminder again that we can't view the mind and body in isolation. The research is clear. They are inextricably linked.

The pain of that memory needs acknowledgement and eventual release.

I'm trained in a model of trauma therapy called EMDR (eye movement desensitisation reprocessing). If I'm working with someone with severe trauma using this model, on occasion it can be difficult for that person to access their traumatic memory or memories. Sometimes when this happens, they can access those memories through physical bodily sensations instead.

I once treated a young woman who had been tortured in her home country because of sexual orientation (same-sex sexual activity is illegal in 69 countries). She had all the symptoms of severe PTSD but struggled to recall the details of her experiences. During treatment she started to cry and protect her arms. She was clearly in pain. After a while she began to settle, and we finished the session.

When I asked her about protecting her arms while crying, she looked a little puzzled. She had no recollection of doing that. Then she rolled up her jumper to reveal multiple cigarette burns. While her mind couldn't remember these being inflicted upon her, her body remembered and her distress was expressing itself in the pain she was feeling on her arms, a reliving of the pain she'd felt during torture. Her trauma was manifesting itself physically.

Granted, this is an extreme example. But I use it to demonstrate how, if you are holding on to negative emotions or not dealing with issues in your life, they can get held in the body. This will create discomfort and lead to physical health problems. Research shows that many (not all) physical health issues have some psychological component. This doesn't mean the physiological symptoms aren't real; they are very real. But it's always worth bearing in mind the role psychological difficulties like stress, loss, emotional pain and trauma have to play in bringing about physical health issues in those already at risk, or exacerbating pre-existing symptoms.

Which takes us to your daily body scan. Ask the same question of your body that you asked of your mind, staying seated with your eyes closed. *How is my body today?*

Allow your mind to scan your body, head to toe, simply noting what you find there. Is there tension? Does it hurt anywhere? Maybe you discover an unexpected ache or tingling. It's all fine, whatever you discover, because it's better to be aware than unaware.

Again, I encourage you to maintain your sense of openness, curiosity and compassion. If you do discover an issue with your body, this will inform how you treat your body for the rest of the day.

For now, though, you are simply acknowledging your body: *I hear you. I feel you. I'm here for you.* The therapeutic actions throughout your day will facilitate the release of your pain and help you to understand what it is your body is trying to tell you. But we'll come to those.

WHAT'S MY MIND DOING?

Finally, you want to briefly check in on your mind's activity. *What's my mind doing today?*

Is there lots of activity? Are your thoughts jumping around? Is there a negative script running through your head today? Remember, don't engage with your thoughts. You are simply scanning the landscape of your mind to see what's going on, nothing more. As always, stay open, stay curious, stay compassionate. You're saying to your mind, *I hear you. I see you. I'm here for you.* You will be amazed at what you discover.

When I have a busy mind, I keep it simple with

my check-in and remind myself that it's just a stormy day. I know that I can take actions throughout my day that help quieten the storm, and that's enormously reassuring.

There you are. The first of your ten minutes of daily therapy is complete. Together with a helicopter view of how you are emotionally, physically and psychologically today, you'll likely have discovered masses of new information about yourself – information that you might not have been aware of until now. Isn't it incredible that just one minute can achieve that? Compare this with the mechanical responses we offer to people asking how we are – usually a version of:

- *Fine*
- *All good*
- *Not bad*
- (Or, if you're Irish, *Could be worse*)

They offer no insight into ourselves at all!

Now we move on to the second minute: responding to what you've discovered during your check-in.

MINUTE 2: WHAT DO I NEED TODAY?

When it comes to self-care and self-compassion, as I've said before, people can get twitchy. I see this a lot with my clients. They look a little suspicious and uncertain when either is mentioned, as if I've suggested something weird and wacky. But self-care and self-compassion are just modern-day rebrandings of 'taking care of oneself', something hundreds of more enlightened cultures and communities have been doing successfully for millennia.

More specifically, I view self-care as the *practical* act of caring for yourself, and self-compassion as the *attitude* that comes with it. While one can happen without the other (I can care for myself practically but still be treating myself appallingly in my mind), that should be avoided. Care and compassion need to work hand in hand. I call this *carepassion*: the act of caring for oneself compassionately.

I'm fascinated by our reluctance to be kind and compassionate to ourselves. Being kind to yourself, certainly in Western cultures, is commonly considered to be selfish, egotistical, unfair to others or a sign of weakness. Let's set the record straight: this is absolutely not the case. Treating yourself with kindness and compassion, both in body and mind, improves the wellbeing of the people around you, as well as your own. Scientific research into compassion-focused therapies, mindfulness and neuroscience all indicates that self-care and self-compassion are essential if we want to function well. They are not luxuries.

Based on the discoveries from the first minute of your self-therapy, I now invite you, in the second minute, to ask yourself what you might need today and how can you respond with a *carepassionate* approach to your emotions, body and mind.

WHAT DO I NEED EMOTIONALLY TODAY?

The simplest way of thinking about how best to respond to your own emotional needs is to consider how you'd respond to a distressed child. Most people, when they see a child crying, upset, frightened or vulnerable, will seek to comfort and soothe that child. It's an innate primal response. And that's exactly how we should try to respond to our own emotions (particularly difficult ones) when they arise.

Whatever emotions you've discovered during your check-in, try now to simply ask those emotions, *What do you need?* Allow a moment for the emotion to speak. It may be that an image, a word, a memory, a sound or even a song comes to mind. Clients often describe gaining valuable insights when they follow this process. Here are some examples of needs that arise:

- **Sadness**: I need rest. I need release. I need to be heard. I need to stop.
- **Anger**: I need this to change. I need to be understood. I need to express this.
- **Fear**: I need to feel safe. I need to know I'm not alone. I need to know everything is OK.
- **Loneliness**: I need company. I need to be understood. I need new people. I need someone to listen to me.

When you have a sense of what needs your emotions are revealing, it's time to decide what acts of *care-passion* might help you care for your emotional self that day.

WHAT PRACTICAL STEPS COULD I TAKE TODAY TO HELP MYSELF EMOTIONALLY?

Consider what would help you find a sense of ease and comfort. Here are some ideas for practical steps you could take to soothe yourself:

- Rest
- A day away
- Lunch with a friend
- A walk in the park
- Watching a film
- Cooking a favourite meal

HOW WILL I TREAT MY EMOTIONS TODAY?

Will you go easy on yourself? Will you talk to yourself calmly, and with kindness and acceptance? Will you drop the judgement, criticism and harshness towards yourself?

Notice how the emotions begin to settle. And they do so because they have been given permission to be seen, to be heard and to be as they are. They have been accepted and cared for with compassion by you. It may be that this has never truly happened before. You and your emotional self are now aligned. This is a powerful way to live.

WHAT DOES MY BODY NEED TODAY?

When you check in with your body, whatever you uncover there, it's important to respond to it. You are asking your body, *What do you need?*

Here are some examples from clients who described strong physical symptoms, and what those symptoms revealed about their needs:

- **Pain**: I need release. I need freedom. I need to get away. I need to let go.
- **Tension**: I need to relax more. I need space. I need to express this.
- **Tingling**: I need reassurance. I need some clarity. I need a plan. I need to find ease.

When you have a sense of what your body may need, it's time to decide what acts of *carepassion* might help you care for your body that day.

WHAT PRACTICAL STEPS COULD I TAKE TODAY TO HELP MY BODY?

Whatever your mobility status, some form of action could help unlock the negative energy that's held in your body. I believe the act of moving creates flow that helps unlock areas of 'stuckness'. Here are some ideas for practical steps you could take to soothe yourself:

- Exercise
- Stretching

- Yoga or Pilates
- A walk or a run

HOW WILL I TREAT MY BODY TODAY?

Will you go easy on yourself? Will you treat your body gently, and with kindness, and acceptance? Will you drop the judgement, criticism, and harshness towards your physical self? Will you fuel your body with the nutrients needed to support your health?

Again, when you implement these actions, notice how the body settles. And it does so because it has been acknowledged as it is. It has been accepted and cared for compassionately by you. It may be that this has never truly happened before. You and your body are now aligned. This is also a powerful way to live.

WHAT DOES MY MIND NEED TODAY?

The human brain, like every organ in the body, can sometimes be overworked. It needs time to rest, reset and recover. If you don't create space within the day for this to happen then your brain will soon become exhausted. Taking care of your mind is as essential as taking care of your body.

It is worth remembering that your brain is like a sponge. It is absorbing all the content of your day.

It takes in all your experiences. It responds when you overthink. It activates your 'threat' mechanism when you're in stressful situations. In short, it will keep working unless you instruct it to pause. Techniques such as meditation and breath work are powerful because they can act as a means of instructing the brain to pause or slow down. They create equilibrium. But you don't have to use meditation or breath work – anything that helps create a sense of calm and space in your day is good.

WHAT PRACTICAL STEPS COULD I TAKE TODAY TO HELP MY MIND?

Each day perhaps consider the following, alongside meditation and breath work, if those work for you:

- Rest for your mind (reading for pleasure, a favourite TV programme or film)
- Minimising stress and pressure
- Feeding your mind nurturing information (motivational podcasts, a documentary, a TED Talk, a non-fiction book on a subject of interest)
- Spend time in green spaces (remember that the research highlights the benefits of nature for mental wellbeing)

- Eat healthy foods that promote a healthy brain (there is an abundance of information online from nutritional experts about the positive impact of nutritionally dense food on mental wellness)
- Talk kindly to yourself (critical self-talk creates distress)

Remember: your mind is the epicentre of everything. Maintenance isn't a luxury, it's an absolute must.

HOW WILL I TREAT MY MIND TODAY?

Will you go easy on yourself? Will you treat your mind gently, and with kindness and acceptance? Will you drop the judgement, criticism and harshness? Will you give your mind time to reset and recover?

Notice how your thoughts begin to slow, and how their tone becomes gentler and more compassionate. Acknowledge how your thoughts have more clarity and are more helpful in nature. They make sense. Your mind has been accepted and cared for compassionately by you. It may be that this has never truly happened before. You and your mind are now aligned. This is a powerful way to live.

MINUTE 3: GRATITUDE AND INTENTION

Our brains are hardwired to look for problems. Neuroscientists have estimated that around 60 per cent of our thoughts are negative or fearful in nature. That's a lot of negative thinking! But the challenge is that our brain thinks it's helping us out. It's programmed to prepare for the worst in order to assist you in avoiding harm or danger. Sometimes this will prove useful. But often it has no purpose, apart from creating psychological distress.

The good news is there is a simple antidote to this: gratitude and intention.

Both can help flip the brain into a healthier adaptive way of thinking that will completely change your day.

GRATITUDE

Let me start by saying that I haven't always been a fan of gratitude as a concept, and I'll explain why. I practise meditation daily. Many years ago, I had a teacher who talked lots about the importance of gratitude. But he always made me feel guilty. He would often state that whatever problems anyone in the class was having, they were nothing compared with what others in the world were experiencing. He would then list natural disasters, countries in conflict or a tragic news headline at the time. This would be followed by an instruction to recite a mantra: *I have much to be thankful for.* And, in turn, I'd think to myself, *Shame on you, Owen!*

One evening after class, I noticed a woman from the class sitting on a wall close to the studio. I could tell she was crying. I tentatively approached to check she was OK. She wasn't. Interestingly, she was also experiencing a sense of shame that she wasn't feeling grateful for all the good things in her life. She was deeply sad, and gratitude wasn't high on her agenda.

As we talked, she told me about her 21-year-old son who had been killed the previous year in a motorbike accident. She was in the depths of grief, and was trying to work her way through the enormous sense of sadness and loss. She felt guilty that she had forgotten about the plight of others.

But she hadn't forgotten. Her grief had simply temporarily clouded her ability to empathise with others' pain.

I think it's important, when we employ gratitude, we do so without shame. I completely understand that it can be extremely difficult to evoke feelings of gratitude if you're feeling depressed, anxious, lonely, bereft or hopeless. And that's 100 per cent OK. The human mind won't automatically produce grateful thoughts at these times because it's too busy producing fearful thoughts! But this is where it gets interesting. Psychological and neuroscientific research indicates that when we step into 'gratitude mode' (even if we don't feel like it or need to force it somewhat), our brain will start to naturally produce more feelgood chemicals such as dopamine, serotonin and oxytocin. In short, remembering what you have to feel grateful for will improve your mood and reduce anxiety, quickly. And the more you do it, the more effective it becomes. I know it sounds simple, but the science is convincing.

So, remaining seated and with your eyes closed, think of three aspects of your life that you are grateful for as part of your third minute of self-therapy, whether that be your friends, family, pets, work, home, finances, health, even the weather that day. Absolutely anything that you are grateful for.

When you have identified the three areas, say them aloud to yourself and repeat them a couple of times if that feels helpful. The research indicates that expressing gratitude using language, even to yourself, consolidates the beneficial impact.

When you have done this, take a few deep breaths

and observe any shifts in mood or emotion. Then let it go and move on to the next stage of your third minute: setting your intention for the day.

INTENTION

We can make any day better by starting it with a healthy intention. Now, having an intention for the day doesn't necessarily mean your intention will be granted. You may set out with an intention to become a millionaire but that doesn't mean it will happen!

Let's revisit the work you did in Chapter 4 on the changes you want to make in your life that will bring you a better future, and the work you did in Chapter 5 around authenticity and living your life with new, more flexible rules, beliefs and values that work for you. When you set out your intention for the day, I encourage you to gear it towards what truly matters to you and makes you feel genuinely happy, connected and at peace, rather than materialistic or ego-driven desires.

With your eyes closed and seated quietly, focus on articulating three intentions for the day ahead. If it's helpful, I'll share with you my intentions today:

• **I will show up and do my best**

- I will look after myself, particularly if I'm feeling overwhelmed
- I will try to be understanding and compassionate with those I interact with today

Your intentions will vary daily but keep in mind that their purpose is to act as an anchor for your day that keeps your steady. If you go off track at any point in the day, you can remind yourself of your intentions and come back to a stable base.

MINUTE 4: GROUNDING

Being ready for your day involves grounding. By this I mean steadying your mind and body. Although this is a short grounding minute, you are free to stay with this exercise longer if you would like to and if time allows.

As you know from your foundation work, your mind is often incredibly busy with lots of thoughts (many of them unhelpful). A busy mind creates stress, and when you're stressed, your body creates more cortisol. This leads to a strong sympathetic nervous system response. That is, your mind and body flip into 'threat mode': they expect danger or harm, so are primed for action. This leads to both a physiological and hormonal reaction that leaves you feeling jittery or on edge.

When you start the day slowing down this process, you send a message to the brain informing it that it doesn't need to be in 'threat mode' all the time. This helps deactivate the flurry of activity that we know as stress or anxiety.

There are many grounding techniques that people use to quieten the mind and relax the body. If you have a particular one that works for you, then use it.

For those new to the concept of grounding I am going to use what I consider to be one of the most effective grounding techniques. I use this technique regularly with clients and I've mentioned it before in my previous books.

HOW TO GROUND

I want to start by stating that grounding takes practice, but once you've done it a few times and gotten the hang of it, it will make sense. I encourage you to use the same routine every day, as this part of the self-therapy process will become your *safe place*.

Remain seated with your eyes closed and follow these three steps:

1. In your imagination, go to a place that represents beauty and peace. (Use the same place every day for a sense of familiarity and safety.) Allow yourself to experience everything you can about this place: the colours, the sounds, the smells, the sensations, the tastes. Gently breathe and enjoy the tranquillity of where your mind has brought you. You are using your imagination to adjust your mindset.

2. When you are relaxed, choose a word that is going to help your mind identify that you've come to your safe place. As before, you're going to use the same word every day. It could be any word, but I tend to find something like 'peace' or 'calm' or 'joy' works for my clients. Simply say the word aloud to yourself a few times. You are using language to reinforce a calmer state.

3. Finally, as you sit in this place of peacefulness, simply use your hands to tap each thigh alternately, left to right in a *slow* rhythm. A fast rhythm will not be helpful. You can do this for 20 to 30 seconds. You are using a technique called bilateral

stimulation. Essentially, your imagination has gone to a calm place and your chosen word reinforces that. The act of tapping while you are practising this technique is a further physical reinforcer. It sends a message to the brain that you don't need to be in 'threat mode' anymore. The steady tapping rhythm creates a sense of ease and facilitates the grounded feeling.

When you've finished, open your eyes and reorientate yourself.

The **ready** stage of your daily self-therapy is complete and you are now ready to face your day, whatever it brings.

You have, in four minutes:

- Checked in with your emotional state and the state of your body and mind
- Figured out what you need for the day
- Practised gratitude
- Grounded yourself

You will come back to your daily self-therapy practice for three minutes in the early afternoon. This will be the **steady** section of your day. It will help keep you strong, focused and on track.

CHAPTER 7

STAYING *STEADY*

This chapter will focus on therapeutic techniques to keep you steady. While your morning practice was aimed at setting you up for the day, this part of your therapy is a leveller. It will keep you on track and help you deliver your authentic self for the remainder of your day. It takes three minutes to do but as before, if you have nothing else that requires your immediate attention, then feel free to spend a little more time with your practice.

It's been well documented that few people take breaks in their day to focus on mental wellness. As we know from earlier chapters, it's easy to fall into the trap of keeping going until we're exhausted. And when you're exhausted, it's also easy to fall back into bad habits.

But mind maintenance and self-care are essential, as we know from our foundation work. It's our responsibility to stop and make sure our minds are in a healthy place and that we're looking after ourselves. This is what the next three minutes of self-therapy will focus on.

Sometimes we can have the best intentions for our day. But it doesn't always go to plan. Setbacks, interruptions, conflict, illness, late trains, irritating people, unreasonable bosses and traffic jams can all play a part in changing the outcome of the day.

I am reminded of a client called Meera, who would often fall victim to this. She would start her day with meditation practice. Then she went to the gym. She meditated again during her tea break and employed many well-known self-help techniques throughout her day. However, none of this, I noticed, prevented her day from becoming 'terrible'.

When we explored this, I discovered Meera's job as a surveyor was competitive and highly unpredictable. As we mapped out the deterioration of her day, it was often linked to how she was thinking and consequently behaving. When a deadline for a project shifted, she would begin to think, 'I can't cope, I'm going to fail.'

When a colleague criticised her work she would think, 'I'm not good enough,' and 'I look like a fraud.' The problem was that Meera would heavily engage with these thoughts (because they were connected to her belief system, a concept you'll remember from your foundation work). It didn't stop there. When Meera fell into her thinking traps, she also fell into the trap of their related unhealthy behaviours. She would become argumentative with colleagues, then withdraw from them. Consequently, she would often feel isolated. This pattern would then carry on at home with her family.

Meera understood the *theory* of therapy but wasn't putting it into practice. She was going through the motions of meditation, and from the outside it looked like she was doing everything she was supposed to be doing, but she needed to really *engage* with the work to change her thoughts and behaviours, then maintain those changes. She was addressing the top layer of the cake, which you may remember from earlier, but wasn't making the changes that were needed to the middle and bottom layers.

For most people, bad days are more often a result of emotional responses to events than the events themselves. This is of course excluding more serious incidents such as bereavements, bad accidents, tragedies, etc., which will naturally evoke justifiably strong emotional reactions.

Similarly, the types of *behaviours* we engage in as a response to events can often have more of a negative effect on our day than the events prompting those behaviours. Healthy behaviours tend to lead to healthier days and vice versa.

This **steady** stage of your daily therapy will have three areas of focus over the three minutes. I encourage you before you start to take a separate moment to practise the grounding technique taught to you in the **ready** section of your work. This will get you into the right headspace before you begin.

I also want to encourage you to carry out these three minutes outdoors and while moving – for instance, during a walk. If this is difficult due to any physical limitations, I encourage you to sit outdoors or at least have a view of the outdoors. I also suggest you go somewhere quiet and away from distractions, ideally close to nature. There is lots of research indicating that even short walks in green spaces help reduce anxiety, lower blood pressure and promote a greater sense of wellbeing.

Your morning practice was seated with eyes closed. This is more 'active therapy'. The act of movement while focusing on your three areas will add a greater energy and momentum to your practice. It will also encourage you to step outside of the normal routines of your day. Habits change when you do new things.

The three areas of focus are:

MINUTE 5 | Tweaking thinking traps and unhealthy behaviours

MINUTE 6 | Healthy behaviour review

MINUTE 7 | Random act of kindness

I want to remind you that *you* are the therapist here, and you are engaging with *your* wisdom and insight to manage your own vulnerabilities or weaknesses, both of which *you* will understand better than anyone else.

Remember that every minute you engage with this process brings you a step closer to a healthier perspective. You're retraining your brain, creating new neuropathways that enable your mind to function in more flexible ways. This isn't just a three-minute walk or time outside. This is an intensive three-minute intervention that will shape your day.

MINUTE 5: TWEAKING THINKING TRAPS AND UNHEALTHY BEHAVIOURS

Now that you've stepped out of your day and grounded yourself, let's review your day so far, bringing your awareness to any tricky moments you've experienced.

As you reflect on the details of the events, ask yourself: how did I respond to that, emotionally? What negative thinking patterns were present? These could be, for example, assuming the worst, making assumptions based on what you think others are thinking (but probably aren't), being in self-sabotage mode, believing that you're the problem, or any other negative thought cycles that repeatedly visit you during times of sadness, anger and stress.

Then ask yourself: what underlying beliefs triggered those negative thought patterns in me?

And, finally, ask yourself: what unhealthy or problematic behaviours have I engaged in today? These behaviours could have either been prompted by the negative events in your day so far, and the cascade of unhelpful thinking patterns and underlying beliefs that followed (for example, 'Why did I argue with my boss?', 'Why did I ignore that call from my friend?', 'Why did I arrive late for that meeting?', 'Why was I rude to that person in the shop?'), or they may have caused the negative events.

Flick back to page 114 to see a list of examples of problematic behaviours that you might recognise from your day (although there are many others not listed there).

First, we're going to look at tweaking your thinking traps.

To do this, we're going to revisit the technique we learnt in Chapter 5 for reprogramming negative thought patterns.

Consider: what's the evidence to support your negative thoughts? You'll usually find there is little or none. Then: what helpful alternative thoughts can you replace your unhelpful thought with? Finally: it's time to let go of that unhelpful thought.

I'd like to recount this scenario, as experienced by a client of mine, Jake, which feels like a useful example at this point.

Jake has plans to meet a friend for lunch and they don't turn up. To make matters worse, he spots a post on social media showing his friend having lunch with another friend. He is disappointed and furious.

In the heat of the moment, Jake messages his friend (using a few choice expletives), saying he doesn't want to see him again and that their friendship is over.

Jake has been triggered by what he perceives to be a rejection from his friend, which has activated a host of negative thoughts and underlying beliefs Jake tends to revert to when faced with challenging experiences.

His thought patterns at the time of the event are:

- Why would he do that?
- I must be a rubbish friend
- No one cares about me
- I'm going to end up alone
- I hate him for doing this
- I'm a loser

And so on.

His underlying beliefs are:

- I must have disappointed him. I'm a disappointment
- This must be my fault
- People always reject me
- I'm not good enough

As you would expect, this experience impacts negatively on the rest of Jake's day.

Fast forward to later in the day, and Jake's friend comes to see him at home. He is baffled by the text and doesn't understand why Jake is angry with him. He shows Jake a text that he had received from him earlier in the morning that read, 'Can't make today, let's rearrange for next week.' Jake intended to send this text to a work colleague to cancel a meeting and mistakenly sent it to his friend, who made alternative plans for lunch!

None of Jake's thoughts or interpretations were accurate. In psychology we call this 'cognitive misinterpretation'. It causes drama and many problems for people. It's incredible the stories our minds can produce. Many of us have the potential to write blockbuster movies!

Stop for a moment and consider how often you misinterpret others' words, gestures, facial expressions and behaviours every day. Consider also how much distress this causes if you don't stop to examine whether your initial assumption is true or not.

Jake could have called his friend to clarify the situation or recheck his messages. He could have factored in the history of a long-standing loyal friendship. But when he was triggered, he fell into the trap of a highly emotive response.

It is your responsibility, during this part of your practice, to be aware of where your thinking is at and of what amendments you can make to improve those thoughts. A bad day can be transformed instantly.

Next, we're going to consider how we can respond better in the future to events triggering unhealthy behaviours. Because it's natural and normal that other people and circumstances will continue to trigger you after this point, and you can't stop those triggers. But you *can* learn to respond better.

Ask yourself the question: *What would a more helpful, flexible response be?*

I'm aware that many of your automated negative behavioural responses have likely been part of your life for a long time. Changing these behaviours takes daily practice. But the more you can challenge these behaviours, the more progress you will make. Remember: every time you substitute a negative response with a healthier response, you change your neuropathways.

For example, maybe you have the same argument with your partner or housemate again and again where they are upset you haven't washed the dishes (I think we've all been there). They feel you're not respecting them. You react strongly with something hurtful and they become extremely upset. The atmosphere is tense.

Later, during self-therapy, you reflect, and recognise that some old behaviours were playing out. You were avoidant and self-focused in the first instance. When this is pointed out to you, patterns of anger, projection and defensiveness emerged. You made the other person the problem.

The reality is they aren't. They have held up a mirror to you, reflecting your weaknesses and imperfections back at you. These are hard to accept. Even harder is the shame of someone else seeing those imperfections. So it's easier to fight back. I wonder how often something like this happens in your day. In all our days! We are often at war with others without fully understanding why we feel so hurt and angry, often seemingly disproportionately so.

But I digress. Back to the dishes. What would a healthier psychological response look like? Let's rewind. You haven't done the dishes, your partner or housemate has gotten upset. They say you're not respecting them.

At this point, your initial response is to be angry that your partner or housemate has challenged you and drawn attention to one of your weaknesses. But before you respond and do even more damage to your relationship with someone you care about and want to enjoy spending time with, you allow yourself a moment to pause. Perhaps you flag with the other person that you are taking a moment and will come back to them. This gives you the physical and mental space to reflect without your partner or housemate feeling stonewalled, and leaves the lines of communication open. In pausing, you notice that your partner or housemate is clearly upset.

You ask yourself two questions:

1. **What's going on with me now?**
2. **How can I respond well to this?**

A moment's brief reflection helps you realise that you have been unreasonable, and that you are being avoidant and a little selfish. Acknowledge this to the other person and assure them that you will work on it. They respond calmly and say thank you. You then do the washing-up.

War has been avoided.

This is what I mean when I describe healthy responses and psychological flexibility. You have acknowledged, taken responsibility, and reacted respectfully. The difference in outcome is immense. Your day is calmer and more peaceful.

I know you may now be thinking, 'But these arguments can happen so quickly. How do I stop this?' The answer is simple. Always allow space for the red mist to dissipate. Rather than over-engage and react, you are going to quieten your mind and slow your responses so you can work out what's going on. Then you can offer a considered, open, flexible response rather than a defensive reaction. The outcome will unquestionably be better.

I'm reminded here of a flight I took a couple of years ago. I was directed by a staff member into the wrong line when boarding the plane. I was in the first-class line, and I had booked economy. It was a busy flight, and as I was nearing the door I realised the error. My realisation that I'd made a mistake that couldn't be corrected without me going to the back of an extremely long line, which in turn might lead to my luggage being put in the hold and getting lost (this had happened before), triggered a strong emotional reaction in me: fear of being reprimanded and humiliated in front of the other passengers. I then noticed a staff member walking towards me, and I was aware that my behaviour was about to become defensive and potentially argumentative. I was in 'fight' mode.

I paused for a second, noticing that there was a strong reaction going on for me. I immediately decided to switch modes. As the staff member approached, I smiled at her and explained I realised I was in the wrong line. Switching modes put me in a calmer headspace and meant I was able to think clearly enough to come up with a solution: asking the flight attendant if she wanted me to wait until the first-class passengers had boarded. She thanked me and looked relieved (I think she was expecting an argument). I stood aside and waited a few moments.

Shortly afterwards, I boarded the plane and proceeded to turn right towards the economy section. As I approached my seat a cabin crew member tapped me on the shoulder and asked me to follow him. They were upgrading me to first class!

One simple decision to be mindful of my reactions and consciously decide how to behave led to a very positive outcome. The only downside was that the flight was only five hours. I don't like flying much, but I didn't want that flight to end!

Healthy behaviours contribute to healthy outcomes. This part of your practice, where you consider healthy alternative responses to tricky situations you've encountered in your day so far, will help bring about more positive outcomes in the remainder of your day, and on subsequent days too.

MINUTE 6: HEALTHY BEHAVIOUR REVIEW

Cognitive behavioural therapy is a type of therapy which supports the view that our behaviours directly impact our thoughts and emotions, and all three – emotions, thoughts and behaviours – are linked.

For the same reason, CBT also supports the idea that actions – as in, positive behaviour changes outside of therapy sessions – are just as important as talking within therapy sessions when it comes to improving our psychological wellbeing. Studies on depression indicate that people don't improve with cognitive interventions alone; they need to be active and engaging with everyday life. And this is exactly what my approach is all about. Therapy *must* be about more than talking. In my view, it is utterly pointless to look at thoughts, emotions and psycho-logical processes unless you are also willing to change your behaviours.

In my years of clinical experience, I've noticed that behavioural changes are sometimes disregarded by clients in therapy. Desires, promises and aspira-tions can be expressed, but are they followed through with actions? Rarely, unless those actions are explic-itly encouraged in therapy sessions. So let me tell you what I tell them: if you aren't prepared to change your daily behaviours, then I'm not going to be able to help you. It sounds harsh, but it's true.

With that in mind, let's move on to the second minute of your outdoor practice.

I'd like you to consider what behaviours you've engaged in today that have activated you, spurred you on and made you feel positive. That could be jogging, going to a book club, learning to dance, walking in nature, meditating, painting, swimming, volunteering, or any number of other activities that represent 'engaging with life' for you. (As an aside, I have witnessed clients – such as Philomena with her gardening – making incredible transformations after integrating some of these behaviours into their lives, where previously they'd done very little to engage with life.)

Here are some questions to consider when reflecting on these positive behaviours:

- What have you done today in relation to personal fitness?
- How active, within your capabilities, have you been?
- Apart from daily routine, what other healthy activities have you engaged in?

- What have you done today that has physically or mentally stimulated you?
- How engaged are you with life today?
- Have you engaged in any behaviours today that are detrimental to your wellbeing? (e.g. excessive alcohol consumption, recreational drugs, excessive or nutritionally poor or too little food, unsafe sex or sex that doesn't make you feel good, compulsive or excessive spending)

Depending on your routine, your response will likely vary day to day. But the idea is, over time, to become aware of your behaviour generally and whether it needs to change.

Which takes us to your commitment to more positive behaviours for the rest of the day. Consider the following questions, and let the answers guide you towards a more healthy and active rest of day:

- What's my plan and commitment for fitness today?
- When can I find the time to do something active, within my capabilities?
- What can I do today that feels healthy and activates me?

- How can I stimulate myself today in a healthy way?
- How do I engage more with my life today?
- What behaviours do I need to drop today that don't support me?

Remember, this part of your practice is helping you regain a sense of control in the middle part of your day. Even if the day hasn't gone well so far, this healthy behaviour review enables you to do something about that. You are the master of your behaviours. Your behaviour is not the master of you.

MINUTE 7: RANDOM ACT OF KINDNESS

I deliberated long and hard about whether to include this in your daily practice.

While the concept of 'acts of kindness' is alluded to within some therapy models, its origins are in Eastern spirituality. Despite that, it seems we have a tendency, when we hear the words 'kindness', 'self-care', 'compassion', etc., to perceive these ideas as a little fluffy or even sanctimonious. But the type of kindness I'm talking about is more complex, nuanced and challenging (particularly in the moment) than a hashtag. Which makes sense, seeing as it's about more than just what we say in person and online – it's about changing our behaviour. (This pertains to my earlier point about actions speaking louder than words.) Anyone can use nice words, but it's actions that count.

In the spirit of honesty, my reluctance to use the word 'kindness' results from the word's common association with both social media and religion in modern society. I'm sure you're already familiar with the hashtag #bekind. While the underlying message is positive, this hashtag crops up again and again in toxic Twitter threads, and is often used inconsistently to defend unkind and bullying behaviour.

The idea of kindness is approached similarly by some religions. As I've spoken about before, I was raised a Catholic, but despite priests and bishops preaching about 'loving your neighbour' (i.e. loving everyone, no matter their creed, colour, beliefs, etc.), and everyone being created equal, the Catholic Church hasn't historically been kind to everyone. They marginalise many. Their words and actions don't always match. I don't want to get into an attack on religion or churches, because they also do some great work. My point is kindness and compassion must be for *everyone*, they should mean something and they aren't words that should be just bandied about.

However, if integrated thoughtfully into our lives, kindness can be a powerful therapeutic force for positive change. I'll explain more.

When we struggle as human beings, it is natural to turn in on ourselves. We can become introspective, self-focused, isolated and less interested in the needs of others. It's a form of self-preservation. Sometimes this might serve a healthy purpose during a time of recovery or rest. But if it becomes a longer-term pattern, it's problematic. It can exacerbate low mood, anxiety and general negative patterns. We know from research that an act of kindness towards another increases our sense of wellbeing. This happens for a few reasons. Every time you perform an act of kindness, you:

- Get a chemical hit of dopamine, serotonin and oxytocin (the feelgood hormones)
- Feel connected to other people
- Break patterns of introspection
- Feel valuable and have a sense of purpose (i.e. helping another person feel better)
- Feel like you're involved in working towards a common goal with other people to achieve the greater good

For most of us it's easier to be kind to those close to us as we have established relationships. It's also easier to measure the impact of that kindness. And while I believe any act of kindness is a good thing, I also believe random acts of kindness towards those we may not know or be close to have greater power than acts of kindness towards those we know well.

What do I mean by that?

Those acts of kindness towards people we don't know have more of an impact upon the *giver* of kindness – you – than the recipient *because* they are that little bit harder. The difficulty in performing that act of kindness makes the act itself more selfless, and when we are selfless, something incredible changes within us. We surpass our troubles. We momentarily forget we are in pain. Deep down, we know we have contributed to the greater good. We activate self-healing.

This is why I ultimately decided to include random acts of kindness into your daily therapy.

Let's move on to how you'll be integrating a random act of kindness into your self-therapy and your day.

Within this moment, take time to reflect on what random act of kindness you could commit to today, and how you will go about it. I'm not suggesting grand or expensive gestures like paying off someone's mortgage or buying them a car. Instead, consider how you can make a difference to someone's day by showing them you're thinking of them. This could mean buying the homeless person on the street a sandwich, making a colleague a cup of tea because they look sad, giving way to a car trying to pull out, smiling at someone who looks isolated, speaking to someone who looks lonely, calling someone you know who is struggling, or cooking an elderly neighbour some dinner. Take inspiration from what brightens *your* day.

And the purpose of this minute in your practice isn't simply restricted to thinking about what act of kindness you'll perform that day. It's also about reminding yourself of the power of random acts of kindness not only to others, but to yourself too.

Kindness isn't just a trend or a hashtag. It's a lifestyle choice. It's therapy. It's an act of rebellion.

The **steady** stage of your daily self-therapy is complete, and you are now ready to face the rest of your day, whatever it brings.

You have, in three minutes:

1. Done an inventory of your emotionally challenging moments so far today, and identified the negative thinking patterns, underlying beliefs and unhealthy behaviours that were present

2. Formulated a plan of action for when you experience other similar situations that trigger those thinking patterns, beliefs and behaviours

3. Reviewed healthy behaviours in your day so far and committed to integrating more healthy behaviours into your day

4. Committed to a random act of kindness

You will come back to your daily self-therapy practice for three minutes in the evening. This will be the **reflect and reset** section of your day. During this, your third and final self-therapy check-in, you'll be exploring the lessons from the day, and letting go of unhelpful thoughts to enable a full night's sleep.

REFLECT AND RESET AT THE END OF THE DAY

D o you ever have moments when you look at your bed, fantasising about getting into it and drifting off to sleep? The thought is so tantalising: no noise, no interruptions, no one needing you (unless you have young children – sorry!). Just rest and sleep. Time to get away from it all for a few hours. It's an escape. It's a time to recharge. It sets you up for the next day.

Every piece of research on sleep highlights its positive impact on our wellbeing. But sadly, not everyone finds sleep easy. Many people go to bed stressed and exhausted. Sleep is often interrupted as the unconscious mind works through all the unresolved issues of the day. Many of the stresses of the day become the stresses of the night, and somehow, in the loneliness of night, they can feel insurmountable. This leads to a heighted state of alert. Sleep isn't fully utilised, and this has a detrimental impact on physical and mental health. People are not ending their day in a healthy way and the consequence is insomnia.

Earlier in the book I mentioned rolling out of bed and autopiloting through the day. We addressed this with your **ready** practice. The same issue presents itself at night-time. Many people roll into bed and don't switch off. It's like sleeping in a car on a motorway with the engine running on full throttle.

For some of us, unless we work through and let go of the day's events, sleep will prove a challenge. We are sleeping with many people, and negative events and situations, in our beds! We are literally 'sleeping with the enemy'.

How many times have you ruminated on your day for hours while trying to sleep? How many times have you got up and out of bed because you forgot to defrost the chicken? How many times have you logged in to your email on your phone because you forgot to reply to someone? How many times have you decided to watch another episode of something on Netflix? (I'm guilty of all of these.)

I worked with a woman several years back who worried a lot about other people's perceptions of her. She described going to bed and replaying the events of the day, trying to figure out if she had offended, upset or disappointed anyone. During one of our sessions, she started to name some of the people she would spend her time thinking about. It came to around twenty people. I remember saying to her, 'That's a lot of people in your head to take to bed every night.'

'It sure is. It's an orgy!' We laughed at that but the point was that there was no space for her to rest or recharge. She was 'on' all the time. And that's not sustainable long term, for any of us.

If this sounds familiar, then maybe it's time for a change.

Which takes us to the final part of your daily practice: **reflect and reset**. Forget your bedtime hot chocolate. If you want to really unwind, it's all about bedtime therapy.

HOW DOES IT WORK?

As with your morning and lunchtime practice, I am mindful of time. And while this practice *is* brief – just three minutes before bed (but not actually *in* your bed) – it is jam-packed with useful content.

(As before, if you want to spend longer on this part of your practice, that's fine, too.) I want to encourage you again to do your one-minute grounding exercise – your psychological stretching – before you start.

If sleeping is an issue, you might want to consider using the grounding technique after your practice too, once you're in bed, to help you drift off to sleep.

For this part of your daily practice, I suggest you find a space where you won't be interrupted, either in your bedroom or somewhere else that's quiet. But, as I say, not actually in bed. The reason why I say to avoid doing your practice in bed is because you risk falling asleep, and you don't get all the benefits of the therapy, which could potentially have a knock-on effect on the quality of your sleep that night.

For this part of your self-therapy, in the absence of a qualified therapist to speak to, you will be writing all the words you would ordinarily say in a therapy session in a notepad instead. This is your means of 'processing'.

Arrange nearby a small bowl of water, and a towel or tissues. The final part of your practice will be a cathartic exercise to 'wash away' the day, which I'll explain more about later. But don't worry. This isn't going to be anything weird and wacky. It's just something I do myself at the end of a session with a client that I'd like to pass on to the therapist part of you.

Our focus for this third and final session will be on three areas:

MINUTE 8 | Journalling and letting go

MINUTE 9 | Lessons of the day

MINUTE 10 | Cleansing, energising and ending the day

I'll be giving you some things to *think* about, things to *talk* about and things to *do* during this session.

Again, don't worry if you can't do this whole session in three minutes. As with all practice, it will get easier with time, eventually becoming second nature.

Before we begin, a quick cautionary note that is particularly applicable to this, your end-of-day session, but applies to all sessions, day and night.

One of the rules of therapy is that you never work with a client if they are intoxicated or under the influence of drugs or illegal mood-altering substances (prescribed drugs are excluded here). This is because the brain of a person under the influence can't process information properly. I say this to protect and support you, and completely without judgement. Therapeutic techniques are only helpful when all parties are in a sober, rational, receptive state.

MINUTE 8: JOURNALLING AND LETTING GO

There are many ways of journalling but I'm going to suggest a very short, specific approach. I use this approach because it helps my clients extract the nuggets of important information from their experiences, and prevents them from writing long passages of unhelpful ruminative rambling prose that holds no therapeutic value. It also means you don't exceed your allotted three minutes of self-therapy time, and you get a proper night's sleep!

During this first exercise, we'll be identifying the moments of your day that have caused you distress or upset. These can include those moments in the first half of your day that you identified in Minute 5 of your lunchtime **steady** practice, if they're still playing on your mind. Then we'll look at how to let go of these moments.

You may be wondering if revisiting distressing moments from the day is a sensible idea at bedtime. I believe it is. If we don't process and move on from the events of the day, then we carry them with us, which has a damaging cumulative effect.

I'd like you to recollect the stressful or upsetting events from the day in quite a structured way:

1. **Event:** write down an account of what happened, attempting to stay objective and as close to the facts as possible

2. **Interpretation:** write down how you've interpreted what happened, or what you've come away from the event believing

3. **Consequences:** write down what impact your interpretation of the events is having on your thoughts, your emotions, your wellbeing and your ability to fall asleep right now, in this moment

4. **Closure:** write down the thinking traps you've identified that you're falling into, write down the evidence to support your negative thought patterns, write down the helpful alternative thought you're replacing

the unhelpful thought with, and, finally let
go of the negative thought

Here's an example of how this might work in
practice.

Pam has a meeting with a colleague who reports
into her, where she broaches his poor work perform-
ance. This leads to a disagreement where he walks
out of her office and calls her a 'rubbish manager'.
Her actions are justified, but she feels upset. This is
the **event**. Later that evening, Pam writes in her
journal:

Event: Argument with work colleague
Pam worries about this event for the rest of the day.
As she is going to bed, she is aware of self-doubt
creeping in. She notes a belief, 'I shouldn't upset
people,' taking shape in her mind. This is her **interpretation**. Pam writes in her journal:

Interpretation: I can't upset people
She is aware that she is overthinking and worrying,
and she becomes anxious about going to work the
next day. She is also worried that she won't sleep.
These are the **consequences**. Pam writes in her
journal:

Consequences: *Anxiety, insomnia*

She switches into 'therapy-mode' and identifies that she's fallen into her old thinking patterns of people-pleasing and being overly concerned about what others think. She considers the evidence. It was her duty to bring up the quality of her colleague's work, and she is helping neither him nor herself by staying silent. She gets great results at work, she was promoted recently and she gets on well with her other colleagues. She is a good manager. She can rationally deduce that her actions were valid, and she is able to let the event go. This is her **closure**. Pam writes in her journal:

Closure: *Old pattern activated – I can let go. I did the right thing.*

Pam's situation is typical of what plays out in many of our day-to-day lives. We do the 'right' thing but then self-doubt, self-blaming, or self-deprecating thoughts based on old rules, beliefs, or experiences emerge. When you can see this dysfunctional pattern for what it is, everything changes. You unlearn old beliefs, discover freedom and strength, and build new foundations. You begin to trust yourself.

It is worth remembering that you are not responsible for how other people react to you. There are moments when it is right to be honest. There are moments when it is right to challenge people. There are moments when you can say no. Your purpose in this world is not to keep everyone happy. Your primary purpose as a human being is to honour and respect yourself. When this happens, life happens from a place of stability and authenticity.

Now you understand the process and the format of this evening's self-therapy, it's time to reflect on and work through the tougher moments of your day. Don't repress them or tell yourself you're not *really* bothered by them, or ignore them and try to push them away. Equally, don't allow them to run rampant through your mind as you lie in bed. Deal with them. This new habit will help you create healthier new patterns, rationally letting go and detaching from that which doesn't serve you well.

When you have completed your journal for the day, read back over each event in turn. Then, one at a time, make a conscious decision to let each event go.

We all carry too much 'stuff' around. We misinterpret, we get stuck in unhelpful thought cycles and we fret way too much. This exercise helps you to break free of that. What a powerful way to end your day and enter sleep.

Before you move on to the next stage of your practice, just pause for breath. Visualise all the concerns and worries of the day drifting away. You don't need to carry them anymore. You're ready to move on to the next stage: extracting the lessons from the day.

MINUTE 9: LESSONS OF THE DAY

Life is offering us lessons all the time. Every interaction, event and experience comes with a useful takeaway. But, if you want to benefit from those lessons, you have to be open to learning them, and you need to know how to see them when they arrive.

When it comes to personal development and growth, there's a lot of unhelpful discourse around these so-called 'lightbulb moments'. This discourse tends to promote the idea that lessons come to us in the form of extraordinary Nirvana-like epiphanies and signs: the bigger, the better.

As a young Catholic boy, I was brought on many pilgrimages to shrines honouring the Virgin Mary. Let me preface this by saying that these pilgrimages bring hope to millions of people, and my intention here is not to be disrespectful of anyone's beliefs. Rather, I tell this story to make a point.

One such shrine was in the Republic of Ireland,

and my late mum would take me and my brothers on a six-hour coach journey to watch the 'moving statue'. The statue was meant to not only move, but cry. We would sit up all night, exhausted, waiting for the statue to move. It was often summertime when we went on these pilgrimages. But it was Ireland so it was cold and wet. As you can imagine, if you had fifty or sixty people deliriously tired, sitting out in the cold watching a statue, then eventually someone was bound to see something moving. And they did.

Not only did the statue move and cry but there were also reports of it waving. The moving statue would also invite a few guests along, including Jesus and some well-known saints. It was quite the celestial celebrity bash.

People would leave elated because they had had signs of 'something bigger'. They believed they were being blessed and gifted with lessons: Jesus saw them, He saw everything they did and did not do, their belief in Him would be rewarded in Heaven, He forgave them, they were good people, they had value. I believed I would catch pneumonia and one day write a book called *The Moving Statue* (watch out for that one). But my point is a serious one: our fellow pilgrims were looking to the extraordinary for an inspiring lesson. But the most powerful lessons are often in the ordinary. They are in the simple moments. They are in moments of silence. They emerge when you listen. They emerge when you see without judgement. They are in the 'cup of tea' moments. They are the stranger who smiles at you at the bus stop. They are a friend who calls when you need it most. They are in disappointment, failure and letdowns. Lessons are everywhere. They are the moments that move you forward, help you understand, prompt decisions and help you find clarity. They are those unexplainable moments when something lands, and suddenly it feels right.

These moments are sadly often lost. In my experience this happens when we:

- Stop listening
- Seek answers in the wrong places
- Close ourselves off to new possibilities
- Forget what matters
- Live on autopilot, not seeing beyond to the greater purpose of our lives

HOW CAN YOU FIND THESE LESSONS?

I want to be clear: the lessons I'm talking about here aren't necessarily practical. They're not the answers to questions like, *How can I make more money? How can I get that promotion? How can I look ten years younger?* These lessons are deeper and are more profound than that. You might learn what makes you truly happy (and that it's not what you expected). You might realise how much a particular person enhances your life, or how much another detracts from it. You might discover how much more resilient your children are than you'd realised, or that they are teaching you just as much as you are teaching them. You may get some insight into your partner's deepest fears and discover that you have the power to allay those fears. A moment of kindness from an unexpected source might remind you that humankind is good. You might realise that you're not being true to yourself in some way.

During the second minute of your evening self-therapy, cast your mind back to your foundation work — your areas of struggle, your story, your rules, your ways of thinking, your emotional and behavioural patterns and what matters to you, and ask yourself this simple question:

WHAT DID LIFE TEACH ME TODAY?

Try to pinpoint the moments when you felt strong emotions. What thoughts were you having throughout the day? Were some old beliefs triggered? Did you, or someone you interacted with, speak or behave in a way that runs counter to your values? Did any moments or events stand out?

Just allow space to pause, and let the information come. Try not to force it too much. The answers will flow if you stop and listen.

I'm going to share with you now the lessons I took from my own practice yesterday in the hope they're helpful.

I was extremely tired going to bed, and I noticed as I checked in with myself that my mood was a little 'flat'. I'd just finished watching a film in which the main character's horse dies. She grieves for the animal deeply. I found it upsetting to watch.

When it came to considering what lessons I could take from the day, I realised that my 'feeling flat' was my own grief. Both my dog and a close friend died a few months ago. I miss them both. My life has been incredibly busy since these losses. My lesson was that I am not giving myself enough space to grieve. This was an important lesson for me to be reminded of.

Life was teaching me. But I would not have been aware of these lessons unless I had created the space to stop for my end-of-day practice.

Lessons can be positive reminders of the import-ance of gratitude and appreciation. Equally they can be signposts to tweaks or changes that need to happen in your life.

Stay open and curious, and let your life teach you. There are many treasures to be found.

MINUTE 10: CLEANSING, ENERGISING AND ENDING THE DAY

You have arrived at the final minute of your daily practice. This is where you will cleanse, energise and close your day. Your day is complete, and you are now ready for sleep before beginning another day.

CLEANSING

This isn't a ritual taught in formal therapy training, but it is popular in healing practices. A supervisor of mine showed me how to incorporate it into the end of my sessions many years ago. He believes that immersion in water enables the therapist to let go of the challenging aspects of work done in the previous session, so they're able to start the next session with a renewed sense of energy and a clean slate.

While I appreciate this is self-therapy rather than

therapy with another individual, I think you'll nevertheless find this ritual valuable. I'll explain how it works.

All you need is a small bowl of water, enough to wash your hands in.

Immerse your hands in the water. As you bathe your hands, visualise cleansing away any negativity, anger and resentment from your day. You are letting your day go.

This end-of-day cleansing ritual is a healthy way to self-soothe, enter 'reset mode' and reinforce the idea that negative influences will not be interrupting your sleep. You are giving yourself permission to let the day go, and this will bring you a sense of peace and contentment.

It's also an act of honour. Cleansing rituals are popular in a variety of cultures all over the world, where they're considered a traditional way of honouring and looking after yourself.

You may have heard the expression, *Namaste: The light in me recognises the light in you.*

You are recognising the light in yourself.

ENERGISING

In this, the second part of the final minute of your daily practice, I would like you to endeavour to connect with something bigger than yourself. Bear with me here. This doesn't have to mean religion, or a god (but it can do). It can mean the solar system, for instance. Looking up at the stars, contemplating the beauty of our world, the miracle – the almost mathematical impossibility – of your very existence, has a powerful effect. It can give you some serious perspective. The knowledge that all your problems are tiny microscopic dots in the context of all of space-time? It's very freeing.

Whether it be karma, fate and destiny, Mother Nature, Wicca, enlightenment, ancient wisdom, energy, the laws of the universe, or simply some unknowable, unexplained and unexplainable higher power, whatever you feel most attuned to, find a way to connect with it.

Why do I ask you to connect with a belief or with something bigger than you? Because it's impossible, and frankly irresponsible in my line of work, to ignore the findings of multiple research papers within the field of psychology which indicate that people with a belief in something, whatever that something is, cope better in times of adversity and manage mental health issues better than people with no belief systems. Some form of spirituality or a belief in an energy source can be a useful psychological tool. (There is a flip side here, of course, when it comes to religion specifically. People who are shamed by their religions tend to struggle *more* during difficult times. Something to bear in mind.)

My interest in energy comes from my years of working with people living with terminal illnesses and approaching death. Many of these people described discovering a sense of peace and contentment after relinquishing control of their journey to God, Allah, Mohammed, Buddha and so on. Outside of religious practices, this is described as trusting in the universe, light, energy, nature and so on. Whatever the context, I have witnessed first-hand how much this has helped people during a time that could otherwise have been very distressing. What is the appeal? What links all of these belief systems together? The relief of being granted permission to let go. The liberating knowledge that you cannot control anything, and your life is in the hands of something or someone else. It's the energy you receive from a source far greater than yourself.

So, whatever helps you go beyond yourself in this moment, I suggest you connect to it and practise the art of handing over control and allowing yourself to be energised. If it helps get you into the right frame of mind, you could start by visualising something awe-inspiring such as a mountain range or the ocean. You could listen to a sound that transports you elsewhere, such as rainfall or birdsong, or a piece of classical music. You could start with a prayer if that's what you'd prefer. It could be anything. The only condition is that you relinquish control to the bigger force, and that you are open to allowing this moment to energise you.

ENDING THE DAY

The **reflect and reset** stage of your daily self-therapy is complete.

You have, in three minutes:

1. Journalled about, and let go of, the moments of your day that have caused you distress or upset
2. Discovered the lessons that life has taught you today
3. Cleansed away the negative aspects of your day
4. Allowed yourself to be energised by a higher source

I'd like you now to pass the final part of your daily practice in absolute stillness and quiet. You are acknowledging the day with the power of silence. You are allowing silence to prepare your mind for sleep. There is nothing to do here. There are no actions. There are no more reflections.

It is time for you to enter a deeper stillness through sleep.

You have woven ten minutes of therapy into your day. This time steadies you. It enables you to cope well with whatever unique challenges your day brings. It allows you to live an authentic, honest life. It empowers you to live more fully.

These ten minutes have the potential to be the most powerful of your day.

Make them count.

CHAPTER 9

WHEN LIFE THROWS A MAJOR CURVE BALL

Most of us know that life can throw unexpected curve balls. One day you're feeling great, and everything is going well. You are happy. The next day, something seemingly catastrophic happens, and everything changes. It could be a bereavement, a breakup, redundancy, a failure, illness, an accident, a tragedy, even a natural disaster. It could be anything. Life is full of endless unexpected possibilities and sometimes they are extremely difficult to manage.

I'm writing this chapter eighteen months since reports of one such unexpected change – a virus called Covid-19 – started filtering into the news cycle. Most of our lives have been interrupted and challenged significantly since the beginning of 2020. Therapy has never been more needed due to the avalanche of uncertainty and chaos this event has caused. It's been traumatic, and I believe we're all going to feel the direct and indirect psychological consequences of the pandemic for a while yet. (This is something I speak to in the second edition of my last book *Ten Times Happier*, where I included a bonus chapter on dealing with trauma. I have coined the term 'post-pandemic stress disorder' to describe the psychological suffering caused by the pandemic.)

Yet, despite curve balls being a constant possibility, it's important to avoid falling into the trap of frantically preparing for them, either psychologically or logistically. Most of the time, life offers a lot of joy. It's a lot more sensible to live in the moment and deal with events should they happen (while working on your psychological flexibility so if they *do* happen, you can cope).

Nevertheless, I want to share with you some quick, high-impact coping strategies for those times of great adversity when your ten-minute daily self-therapy isn't going to cut it, just in case you need them.

I'm going to focus on five areas of adversity that all of us will encounter at points in our lives:

- Bereavement
- Change
- Personal illness or taking on a caring role
- Disappointment
- Times of crisis

The therapeutic principles will remain the same but there are some specific considerations and adjustments that make particular challenges in your life more manageable.

More important than any of these, however, is remembering you have survived crises before, which means you can and do cope. I am simply offering you some additional tools and techniques that may help make those crunch points easier to handle.

BEREAVEMENT

Loss is inevitable in life. We have all lost people we love. We will all continue to lose people we love. And that's how it should be. It is the natural order: life and death.

As I mentioned earlier, the first half of my career was spent in palliative care environments working with people who were terminally ill. A large part of that role involved bereavement support for families after their loved one had died. I became familiar with the impact of loss, but I also became aware that grief impacts different people differently, and it doesn't always look the same from the outside.

I believe pathologising grief (labelling it as a disorder) or suggesting that the grieving process is made up of predictable, easily defined psychological and behavioural 'stages' risks minimising a person's loss by indicating that there is an end point by which time they should no longer be in pain. The idea of 'the stages of grief' can also make grieving people feel isolated or guilty because they're not feeling what they're 'meant' to feel. Grief is not that simple or predictable. Sometimes it can be complex, and people do become stuck, but it doesn't mean there is anything wrong with them or how they're grieving. It simply means someone is hurting deeply and finding it extremely difficult to adjust to a life without their loved one. Bereaved people need patience, time and a lot of understanding. A part of them has died, and that must be honoured.

Apart from my professional experience in this area, I am no stranger to grief personally. Each loss has been different, but all have felt raw. Healing from grief is painful.

This is what I know to be true about bereavement personally and professionally:

- Emotions in the early stages of grief have no order or predictability. Sadness, anger, emptiness, bewilderment – in fact, any emotion – can erupt unexpectedly, like a volcano. All you can do is hold tight and wait until it passes.
- People won't always understand your loss, and their insensitivity is more often linked to a sense of powerlessness than them not caring.
- Guilt is a given. Grief will always raise questions: could I have done more? Should I have seen them more? I believe this is the mind's way of distracting us from the reality that the person in our life has gone. If we think, wonder, doubt ourselves, maybe this cataclysmic event will make sense. And for those of us with self-critical thought patterns, our inner saboteur can have a field day during this time.
- There are no shortcuts to dealing with grief and there is no time limit.
- Love is joyful. But it requires enormous courage, because, in loving, we also leave ourselves vulnerable to losing the one we love. It is the natural order of things.

- The pain eventually eases and it is possible to learn to live without the other person.
- Life goes on, but it can never be the same. And that's OK.

WHAT HELPS?

While there isn't a 'one-size-fits-all' remedy for grief, the work you've done around self-care and self-compassion will be vital at this juncture. Looking after yourself during a period of grief is essential. Many of your physical and psychological resources will be significantly depleted. The death of someone you cared about is a huge blow. The mind and body need time to adjust.

Besides self-care and self-compassion, here are a few extra tips for how to deal with a bereavement:

- Create as much space and time as possible to allow yourself to grieve.
- Talk when you need to. Grief needs to be processed. Talking enables that to happen.
- Ask for support when you need it.
- Surround yourself with people who allow you to be sad when you need to be.

- Create some flexibility in your routine. It's impossible to go on as 'normal', particularly in the early days.
- Remember, you are not falling apart – you are trying to come to terms with a significant loss.
- Don't be shamed into thinking there is a right or wrong way to grieve. This is a very individual journey.
- When you are ready, try to celebrate the good memories of the person you are grieving.
- Manage your grief one step at a time. Hour by hour. Day by day.
- Remember that you can survive this. You are hurting because you loved.

CHANGE

Our lives are in a constant state of flux. The next change is always just around the corner. But we tend to seek stability, predictability and order. Even adventurous personality types like a plan. And why do we seek stability? You may remember from your foundation work that 'feeling safe' is one of the most important contributors to healthy childhood development. Periods of change can threaten that feeling of safety in children, leaving them feeling unsettled and exposed. And it's the same with adults, particularly when experiences trigger distressing memories of change during childhood. I notice my clients' moods taking a dip or their anxiety rising during periods of transition. In psychology, we refer to these as 'adjustment disorders' but I prefer not to use the word 'disorder' to describe this feeling. I don't think there is anything unusual about struggling in the face of change.

In summary, this is why we seek out routines. They're a survival mechanism. They help us feel a bit more in control.

But the truth is that control is an illusion, because we *don't* have control over life events. Which is why, while it's positive and stabilising to establish routines, we must also embrace uncertainty and live in the now.

I once read a story about a monk who lived in the same monastery for twenty-five years. He was deeply peaceful and content. Every few years the monks would have a new superior who would come along and change some of the routines in the monastery. During one such period of change, the new superior suggested to the monk that he go travelling on a train for a year to experience uncertainty. He wanted him to broaden his perspective away from the monastery.

The monk became very unsettled about this, realising he had built his life around safety, predictability and avoiding challenges. But he understood that he needed to go on this journey.

He did so, and despite the sense of unease it brought, it led him down a path of personal growth. His meditation practices improved. He discovered many new personal strengths. He developed a greater sense of compassion. Interestingly, he never returned to the monastery. He took to life on the open road, fulfilling his duties as a monk in a more nomadic way. He found a new sense of freedom.

And just like the monk, while change (for instance, redundancy, a break-up, a house move, immigration or a new job) can often be at the heart of struggle and make our foundations feel unsteady, it can also be an opportunity for emotional and psychological growth.

The way through these periods of change is to face them courageously, embrace them as adventures, and approach them with excitement and curiosity, knowing there are lessons contained within these experiences if you choose to listen out for them. Who knows? There could be something incredible waiting on the other side.

WHAT HELPS?

As before, the basic principles of therapy and your ten-minute practice apply.

Besides those basic principles, here are a few additional tips for how to cope with big changes in your life:

- Create a sense of 'internal' familiarity by committing to some of your normal daily routines.
- Push yourself to face and get involved with the day-to-day aspects of whatever the change is. This will feel uncomfortable, but that doesn't mean it's wrong. Work at a pace that you can manage without feeling overwhelmed.
- Keep in contact with friends and family who are able to offer helpful support.
- Observe your expectations and be aware that small steps at a gentle pace will be enough to start with.
- Remind yourself that the vulnerable feelings you have may not be directly linked to the change but rather some old memories or beliefs that have been triggered.

- Give it time. Adjusting to change requires patience and a lot of time.
- Safety behaviours are likely to emerge in which you have a sense of wanting to run away from or avoid the change. Be mindful this is simply an anxiety mechanism, and doing the opposite will be more helpful longer term.
- There is no 'right' or 'wrong' way to feel during a period of change. Your experience is your experience. Turn up the self-compassion a few notches!
- Finally, a cliché but one I love: boats aren't built to sit in harbours. Change means you are alive, and your life is moving forward in a new direction. Embrace it as best you can.

PERSONAL ILLNESS OR TAKING ON A CARING ROLE

As a former nurse, I'm very aware of the impact illness and being a carer can have on a person. None of us knows when a period of illness or caring for another will come. But the likelihood is, it will. It's part of life. I will look at how you can manage periods where you yourself are ill, and how you can manage when you're in a caring role separately, as they both come with completely different sets of challenges.

I want to preface this section by saying that when I talk about 'ill health', I mean both physical and psychological. The human body and mind are complex, and sometimes they run into problems. We know from research that the mind and the body are interconnected. They can't be considered in isolation.

Unquestionably, psychological ill health can contribute to poor physical health and vice versa. A person could be ill at home following a heart attack, but also very depressed as a result. A person trapped at home with agoraphobia could have cardiac problems because they aren't able to exercise. We must move on from this antiquated approach of viewing physical and mental health as two separate issues. They are not. And I say that with total confidence, having spent my entire career in both worlds.

When you experience a period of illness, whatever the cause, your life can change suddenly and drastically. Aspects of daily life become temporarily or sometimes permanently interrupted: your social life, work, ability to see or spend time with your family, sex life, income and overall finances, how you spend your leisure time and so on. In short, the disruption to what you can do caused by your illness impacts significantly on your freedom, choices, decisions, interactions and how you feel. These changes can happen slowly too, which brings its own challenges: your quality of life can drop steadily over the course of weeks, months or years, but slowly enough that you barely notice the difference, until you wake up one day and your life is unrecognisable compared with the one you used to live. Whatever your experience of illness, coping isn't easy. You are adapting to living with restrictions and limitations (whether in the short term or longer term – or perhaps you may have no idea how long your recovery is likely to take, and that 'not knowing' can be extremely challenging, too). This doesn't feel fair. Coming to terms with your situation, especially when we're talking about chronic illness, is difficult. But it's possible.

WHAT HELPS WITH ILLNESS?

As before, all the strategies and techniques you've learnt so far throughout this book, as well as your daily ten-minute practice, will help you cope with your illness. But I'd like to also offer some additional thoughts on how to cope specifically with illness, based on my many years' experience working in physical and mental health settings.

But before I go any further, let me first say that some of these suggestions may suit you better than others, depending on your circumstances. Some might even make you feel angry if you don't feel like they're taking into account the unique challenges of your situation. I totally appreciate there can be nothing worse than someone offering advice if you feel they don't understand your illness. I want to reiterate, however, that my sole aim here is to try to support you and bring some sense of ease. If one of the suggestions I've made makes even a little bit of sense, then I encourage you to go with it or at least consider it. Trust my experience and what the research reveals.

Here are my suggestions for what might help psychologically if you're suffering from illness:

- The physical body experiences more pain and more symptoms when the mind is distressed. This leads to the mind becoming *more* distressed. It's a vicious cycle. Focus on using techniques that quieten and relax both mind and body. They'll be enormously beneficial.
- In times of illness, it's essential that you make adjustments to your daily routine and endeavour to be flexible when things don't

go to plan. It isn't possible to go on as normal. Trying to do so creates more distress.

- Compliance with treatments and professional guidance is sometimes crucial.
- Acceptance in times of illness comes with huge challenges. But the research within Acceptance and Commitment Therapy shows that accepting what the situation is rather than what it could be or what it should be can reduce your resistance to the fact of your illness, which has a knock-on beneficial impact overall. I know how difficult this can be in practice but try resisting less. Notice what happens.
- Self-care must be a priority.
- Hope can help. Although not easy, the research shows that opting for a hopeful perspective can improve how you feel. I want to be clear; this isn't inconsistent with acceptance. You can both accept that you're ill and still have hope. Hope means allowing yourself to see possibilities, even if it's just one simple thing. For example, it could be that you are going to try to enjoy your garden, get outside a little more or do one activity every day that you know lifts your

spirits. Your brain chemistry changes for the better when you allow yourself moments of hope.

- Focus on self-soothing. When the going gets tough, dig deep for that compassionate voice that helps you find ease.
- Practise mindfulness. The research is clear that daily mindfulness during times of illness can significantly improve symptoms. There is an abundance of material available online, in books and via in-person or online courses if you want to explore this further.

For any of you struggling now with illness, I send my thoughts and well wishes to you. May you find comfort in some of these words.

CARERS

Caring for someone who is ill, no matter how much you love them, can be exhausting. Not only are you watching someone suffer but, as a carer, you are performing numerous roles practically, physically, emotionally and psychologically, often with little support or recognition.

If you are caring for someone who is ill, I want to acknowledge the rollercoaster that this is for you.

You are doing your best, but it never feels like it's enough. You are tired but feel guilty when you need a rest. You want to be loving and kind but have moments when you are irritated. You want to be understanding but you are tired of listening. You want to be there all the time, but you desperately want a rest. You long for your life back.

If any of this resonates with you, I want to assure you I've heard this from so many other people who were or are in a similar situation to the one you find yourself in now. You are human, and caring comes with personal losses. There is nothing abnormal, unkind or worrying about any of these feelings. Unnecessary guilt may try to tell you that you must be on your 'A game' all the time. It simply isn't possible. You are likely doing your very best and that is enough. If the person you are caring for was caring for you, they would likely be experiencing similar feelings.

We are all human. We get tired. We experience compassion fatigue. We struggle. But despite all of this we keep going and we turn up again the next day. That is the reality for most carers.

I'll say it again because it bears repeating: you are doing your best.

WHAT HELPS IF YOU'RE A CARER?

I won't be overly prescriptive here as each situation varies, but these are psychological strategies that have made the lives of carers I've worked with easier:

• Take breaks and get help. As simple as this sounds, these are probably the most important suggestions I can make. Most carers believe they must do it all, all of the time. You don't have to. There is help available if you seek it. The more rest you have, the more available you will be for your loved one.

• Observe the role of guilt telling you that you are not doing enough or failing. Challenge this internal voice, and recognise that this is an unhelpful and false narrative rather than a fact.

• Talk about your struggles with other carers. It will help you feel understood, and less isolated and alone. Talking to other carers about their own struggles will also help you to be more compassionate towards yourself, as you recognise your challenges in theirs.

• Self-care must be prioritised above your caring role. If you burn out or become exhausted, then you won't be able to help. This is not a selfish act. It's an essential act to enable you to function.

- Keep a journal. Sometimes it will be difficult for you to voice your frustrations or feelings out loud. Journalling every day will help you process and deal with what's going on. Keep a therapeutic focus on thoughts, emotions and reactions.

DISAPPOINTMENT

It's a horrible feeling, disappointment. That sinking realisation in your gut that something hasn't worked out as planned. It could be that you didn't get the promotion you were promised, the new home you set your heart on has fallen through, you didn't get the grades you needed, the relationship you thought would make it to the altar has ended, your IVF treatment has failed or you've discovered one of your children is dependent on drugs. It might not be one single event. Maybe life simply hasn't worked out as you hoped it would. Disappointment is part of life. It shakes our foundations.

I hear about disappointment every day in my office. Sometimes my clients are furious and bitter. I've heard it all:

- 'I can't believe this hasn't worked out'
- 'This is just my luck'
- 'I'm doomed'
- 'Life isn't fair'
- 'Why do good things never happen to me?'
- 'I don't see the point in trying anymore'
- 'I should just give up'

I'm sure everyone at some stage has felt this way. Disappointment when life doesn't go to plan activates a very strong personalised response. In other words, it becomes personal! The world is out to get you. This disappointment must be part of a master plan to push you to the ground. It seems you have been specifically targeted and screwed over by life.

I was recently on the London Underground and we got stuck in a tunnel for ten minutes because of a signal failure. The driver was apologetic and to be fair was providing regular updates. The woman seated beside me was on her way to see *Mamma Mia!* at the theatre with her friend, and they would now be fifteen minutes late and possibly refused entry. I know this because I was listening in on their conversation. She was incensed. How could this have happened? She proclaimed that not only was her evening ruined but the entire weekend was ruined. It got worse. She had lost £80 on tickets, and there was no way she would ever be coming back to London again. It was all a complete disaster. She was going to write to the London Underground and her MP to let them know what a 'shambles' the city's train system was.

I must admit I was slightly tempted to intervene with a little dose of therapy but there was no need. Her friend remained very quiet and attentive during the rant but when it was finished, she spoke (and I paraphrase from memory):

'Love, would you prefer the driver risk our safety so we can go and sing along to *Mamma Mia!*? Why don't you try to calm down? Let's find a nice bar, have a few cocktails and check out the hot guys in town. We can get cheap tickets for the matinee tomorrow and make the best of the evening.'

As soon as she'd finished speaking, the tube driver announced that the signal failure was sorted and we were about to get moving again. Disaster had been averted. Julia (yes, I even caught her name during my eavesdropping) *would* get to see *Mamma Mia!*. Her friend would have to wait until after the show to go to the bar and check out the hot guys.

This moment really stuck with me. Julia was clearly disappointed at the thought of missing the musical. She was immediately triggered, and her negative cognitive processes went into autopilot. I assume that she had patterns of feeling victimised, catastrophising, thinking the worst, not taking into account the positives and personalising life's adversities. Observing her rant was like watching a landslide that just couldn't be stopped. Life wasn't delivering what she wanted and expected in that moment, and she refused to tolerate that. She was creating her own distress.

We all have our own *Mamma Mia!* moments. Some won't be that serious, some will be incredibly disappointing. I don't want to minimise the impact of disappointment. It's healthy to feel and acknowledge disappointment. It's never advisable to push away those feelings. But the problem is getting stuck or falling into the trap of being triggered unnecessarily.

WHAT HELPS?

You already have a host of tools available around managing thoughts, emotions and beliefs. When it comes to dealing specifically with disappointments, there are a few additional psychological tools that could come in handy:

- Become familiar with what disappointment feels like for you and how you normally respond. If you identify that you are easily triggered in certain situations, create space by allocating additional time during and after those situations (insofar as they can be anticipated) to allow your distress to settle.

- Initiate perspective check-ins. How important is this? Are there other possibilities? Is there another way of looking at this?
- Trust the process. If you can't control the outcome, allow yourself to let go of that expectation and just be.
- Remain open to other possibilities. There is a very wise saying: 'When one door closes, another opens.'
- Review your tolerance levels when life doesn't deliver what you want or expect. Life doesn't work the way we think it should. Life expects us to work *with* it. Hard to swallow but true.
- What can this teach you? I truly believe that we learn more from disappointments and setbacks than we do from successes, so long as we keep our minds open enough to hear those lessons. Salvage what you can from the circumstances rather than being paralysed by the disappointment. Many 'successful' people have allowed disappointment to teach them. It is a wise path to follow.

TIMES OF CRISIS

What constitutes 'a crisis' can mean different things to different people. But I am going to define 'crises' as those times in life when your sense of stability and ability to cope are significantly compromised. This could be due to a life event, personal circumstances or feeling like you've 'fallen off the wagon'. Put simply, normal everyday functioning is a real struggle. You might feel overwhelmingly out of control, hopeless, powerless and despairing. There may be times when you have suicidal ideation or intent. Remember, this doesn't mean there is anything 'wrong' with you as a person. It simply means you are unwell. You are in crisis. This isn't just a bad day or a rough patch. And you shouldn't do this alone.

The problem with crisis periods is that a chain of events is set in motion that renders the situation almost impossible to manage (or at least, that's how it feels). Emotional distress is probably highly elevated. Chemically, your brain is likely releasing a surge of stress-related hormones. Accessing rational responses becomes almost impossible. Day-to-day functioning is impaired. Communication becomes difficult. Relationships can feel challenging. It all generally feels like too much, leaving you feeling incredibly isolated.

This isn't a time for therapy or working out patterns. This is a time for seeking help that enables you to return to a place of stability. You can work out what's going on later in therapy.

I often see people in crisis directed to therapeutic services which, at that time, they are unable to engage with. This doesn't mean therapy won't eventually be helpful. It will. But just not yet. It's like sending someone to sea without a life jacket.

There are several steps that will help you to do this, which I'll explain now.

WHAT HELPS?

- Acknowledge that you're overwhelmed and ask for help. I know how hard this can be, but I promise you, when you speak to a professional, they will have seen this a thousand times before. They will understand you are in crisis and will be able to help you. I have provided a list of organisations at the end of this book.
- Don't be afraid to stop or pull back from normal everyday activities that are too much for you.
- This isn't the time to try and work out what's going on, or find practical or logistical

solutions to commitments in your life. Hand this over to others temporarily, if you can. The priority now is getting the right help and support to get you back to a place of stability. I see too many people try to take this road alone. This is not a solo journey – trust me on this.

- Share with a few trusted people close to you that you are in crisis and ask whether they can be your emergency contacts. This way they can carry out the unavoidable duties you'd normally be doing; they can bring food, help with household chores and childminding, let your workplace know you won't be coming in, or just come over and listen, even if it's the middle of the night.
- Medication is sometimes suggested during these periods. In my experience professionally, short term, this can be incredibly helpful. Always discuss with a trained professional the best options for you.
- *Remember, crisis periods are temporary and they do end. You can get through this.*

When I meet a person in crisis, they often say they feel weak or ashamed that they have got to this point. I respond by reminding them that there is no reason to feel shame, and that they are the opposite of weak. The fact that they, and perhaps you if you're in crisis right now, can carry on putting one foot in front of the other when you're feeling the way you do demonstrates enormous courage and strength.

No one chooses to get to a point of crisis. Sometimes life is the real issue. There is no failure or shame in crisis. I see only bravery, humanity and a fellow human being who needs help to stand up again. **If you are struggling to cope, always seek professional help. You can get through this.**

CHAPTER 10

ALL'S WELL THAT ENDS WELL

I started this book by sharing some insights into the world of therapy, and hopefully demystifying it. I want to end it by reinforcing the power of therapy with some real stories of transformation in the lives of my clients. I want to remind you that, whatever has happened, there is always hope. Something good can be salvaged from almost any situation – maybe not straight away, but eventually.

Before I do that, though, a few thoughts on what happens after you finish reading this book.

I'm always struck when I finish reading a book and experience a range of now-familiar emotions:

- Sadness that it's ended
- Loneliness that I won't have the writer's voice or characters with me
- Elation if there's a happy ending
- Frustration if it ends on a cliff-hanger
- Disappointment if I didn't get the ending I wanted
- Challenged if the book has awakened my mind to issues I was previously unaware of
- Angry if characters I liked found themselves in situations that are unfair or unjust
- Inspired to make changes or do something new

You too may experience some unexpected feelings as this book ends, but not just because it's a book. This is a therapy book. Endings in therapy provoke emotions. I think it's important to take a moment here to acknowledge that.

If coming to the end of this book has brought strong feelings to the surface, that's completely understandable and to be expected. You may feel a little sad that a familiar voice is gone. You may feel frustrated that you have work to do. You may feel excited by the prospect of new possibilities. You may feel disappointed that I haven't sorted out all your problems.

The exciting news is that you now know how to recognise, manage and work with these feelings. They aren't abnormal. You are dealing with an 'ending' of sorts and we need to take note of your emotional responses to that. It's an important part of the process in therapy to acknowledge the end of a therapeutic relationship. It's part of the closure process. It helps with a sense of completion.

On the other hand, it may have been the *process* of reading this that was more emotional for you. Remember I said at the start that good therapy isn't fluffy and warm all the time. If it's made you a little uncomfortable or uneasy at points, then that's great (and I mean that in the kindest possible way). I'm doing my job and you are responding. Change is uncomfortable.

Equally, the book will hopefully have awakened thoughts of a better future and discoveries of new strengths. If you realise that you are now looking at life and situations through a different lens, that's great too. Again, I'm doing my job and you are responding.

Consequently, you might realise there are some areas of your life that you want to change. I encourage you to go at a steady, considered pace and try not to change everything at once. Take it one step at a time. The next best step is enough and that's all there is to manage.

I hope the book has challenged you and inspired you to take the time to switch into a therapy mindset. But – and this is the important bit – you will only notice improvements if you commit to this work. I regularly encounter clients who want me, as the therapist, to make everything better for them. It doesn't work that way. It takes work.

In this book *you* are the therapist, and *you* are also doing the work. Reading the book isn't going to be enough. This is a book that requires action long after you have finished reading. But it will be worth it. The more you show up to practise what you have learnt here, the better you will feel. Your life will improve. Try to think of it like going to the gym. The more you apply yourself, the greater the results.

I'm equally aware you might decide that the techniques in this book aren't enough for you. You may want to get professional help with issues that you are finding difficult. You might decide you want to have some one-to-one therapy! And if that is the case, congratulations on getting to that point. If this book has helped you make that decision, then equally, my work is done.

If you decide on one-to-one therapy with another therapist, a few tips. Finding a therapist that's right for you can be like finding a needle in a haystack.

My advice is to ask around. Recommendations from people you know, or from your doctor, will help you identify the right therapist for you. There is also some useful online advice from mental health charities such as MIND and SANE.

It's important that you know what therapy models your therapist is trained in. Ask questions about their qualifications and experience. It is also wise to check they are fully qualified and accredited with a recognised regulatory body. This varies from country to country so you will need to check what those are in your region.

Whatever your experience has been reading this book, it's over to you now. I hope you feel empowered to live a fuller life with the information and skills you now have. I hope that prospect excites you.

But before I say goodbye, as promised, let me share with you a few stories of clients I've worked with who have inspired me. The stories I share with you focus on people who have experienced the worst of times and worked through it. They also learnt to become their own therapist (which, as I said at the start, is always my ultimate goal). They live the principles of this book.

I hope they inspire you as they inspired me. I hope they encourage you to walk this path.

MARGO: THE GLITTER BALL STAYS

Margo came to see me seventeen years after the death of her daughter. She had seen many therapists since the loss of her daughter, and their focus had been on grief or depression. But her level of distress during our introduction raised a suspicion in my mind that something else was going on.

She told me about the loss of her beautiful daughter on holiday. She was 21 and died in a tragic accident. Margo couldn't come to terms with the loss.

By the end of our first session, I had no doubt Margo was grieving her daughter and experiencing secondary mood symptoms, but the missing link soon emerged. She was also deeply traumatised by her daughter's death. There were several traumatic memories including seeing the body for the first time, the funeral and her imaginings of what happened on the day of the accident. She was experiencing PTSD (post-traumatic stress disorder) and met diagnostic criteria for treatment. Trauma that is not processed won't settle until it is treated. (I interject here with a reminder that if symptoms associated with trauma, anxiety or low mood are not improving after two to three months or so of consistent self-therapy and changes to your behaviour, always speak with a professional.)

We focused initially on Margo's trauma during her therapy sessions. Within several weeks Margo was showing improvements. Fast forward to a few months later and she'd booked a cruise holiday with her friend. She came back having had the most incredible holiday and for the first time in seventeen years she felt like her 'life was coming back'. She started to socialise again. She started painting again (a hobby she'd previously loved). Generally, she started to engage more with her life. But she didn't stop there.

Margo's house had been unchanged since her daughter's death, including her daughter's bedroom. She decided to renovate. When she was planning the renovations, she explained to the builders that the bedroom couldn't be touched. It had become a shrine to her daughter, and no one could enter the room. It was also therapeutically representative of how 'stuck' Margo had become.

We discussed this sense of 'stuckness' in therapy. Margo eventually recognised this and agreed to instruct the builders to renovate her daughter's bedroom too. But there was one condition: *the glitter ball stays*. The glitter ball was one of her daughter's favourite possessions. Margo believed it captured the essence of her daughter's fun and energy.

The bedroom is now an art studio. Margo now paints regularly under the sparkle of the glitter ball. She has rekindled the spark in her own life.

Alongside Margo's trauma treatment there were several other therapeutic factors that helped in her recovery.

She discovered that taking time out each day to be her own therapist was important. She realised connecting with people and reconnecting with life was part of her recovery. She discovered that some of her unnecessary guilt was linked to years of unhelpful rules and beliefs. Above all, she realised that facing and dealing with the awful reality of her loss was the only way forward. For years, she has been focused on her own sadness and managing the symptoms of that sadness. Facing the trauma around her loss was her first step towards healing.

I share Margo's story with you because she is someone who taught me a lot about the journey from hopelessness to hope. She also taught me that in the world of therapy, sympathy and platitudes aren't enough. Sometimes the work is challenging and requires us to go to dark places. Often, that is the way through.

Margo's grief and sadness had become a familiar safe place for her to go. During therapy I was gradually moving her away from this, not because we were avoiding the sadness, but because it was preventing her from living.

I don't believe any of us ever truly 'get over' the big losses in our life. We get through. And that's enough and perhaps how it should be.

Margo's journey of seventeen years was a long road. And I reminded her that there would be times when it would feel like she'd been thrown back into the deep end of her grief again. But she now has the insight, wisdom and skills to become unstuck. This is the power of therapy. She is now her own therapist.

So, if you're feeling stuck today in the same sad, angry or despairing thought cycles, there is always a way forward. There is always a glitter ball to be found somewhere in the dark. Margo's story teaches us that.

KYLE: WHY AM I ALWAYS SCARED?

Kyle came to therapy reluctantly. His girlfriend thought it was a sensible idea, so he decided to 'give it a go'. He was one of the people I mentioned earlier in the book who thought therapists and therapy might be 'a bit weird'. Thankfully, I managed to convince him otherwise.

Kyle was experiencing significant anxiety symptoms that he couldn't make sense of. His first question to me was, 'Why am I always scared?'

He experienced worry about most things, most days. He wasn't sleeping well, and he was difficult to be around (according to his girlfriend). He was experiencing generalised anxiety disorder (a diagnostic label that I prefer not to use. Instead, I describe a sufferer as someone who has learnt to worry lots).

Kyle grew up in a small mining community in the north of England. When he was telling me his life story, I noticed his father was absent from most of the story. There was nothing particularly remarkable about Kyle's story. He didn't mention any significant traumas. He described family life as 'normal' (always a giveaway). His school life, university life and social life were all areas in which he appeared to function very well. He simply worried all the time and didn't know how to stop. In short, he was a high-functioning worrier, which is very common.

As I got to know Kyle better, I mentioned to him that I noticed his father was absent from his life story. His father had died a few years earlier. He initially dismissed this as insignificant, saying they simply didn't get on. A few questions later and it was a different story.

Kyle's father was a violent alcoholic for most of his formative years. Kyle and his family members were often physically and verbally attacked by his father during 'drinking binges'. When his father was sober, he was highly critical of everyone in the family. The situation was complicated by his mother, who didn't want anyone outside of the family to know about the drinking or violence. There was a family dynamic of secrecy.

It won't surprise you to know that consequently Kyle grew up with lots of unhelpful beliefs about himself and how to cope with life. His confidence was low. His anxiety was high. He was fearful, but also believed he had to be at his best in life, no matter what. That was his family script. We were able to answer his question, 'Why do I worry so much?'

I share Kyle's story with you because understanding his story was central to improving his anxiety. He had normalised his childhood and his father's behaviours. The reality is that they were a major contributor to his anxiety. Once he understood that, he was able to stop hiding his feelings and looking out for danger all the time, and he could let go of patterns of secrecy and people-pleasing.

He had been 'hard wired' to worry. His daily self-therapy practice involved rewiring his brain to respond with a calmer, more adaptive approach. He had nothing to fear anymore. His brain needed that message to be reinforced.

Kyle learnt the skills of managing his anxiety by using self-therapy, just as we have done together. He practised checking in with his mind, body and emotions every day. He learnt how to 'ground' himself. He was able to challenge unhelpful thinking, and rules and beliefs that didn't serve him anymore. Ultimately his self-therapy taught him how to practise self-care, how to look after himself and how to help himself feel safe.

Several weeks into therapy and daily practice, Kyle began to improve. His anxiety dropped and he reported that his girlfriend had noticed remarkable changes in his behaviour. He worried less. His sleep improved and he was easier to be around. He generally felt happier.

At our last therapy session Kyle brought a small gift to our session. It was a postcard he had found in a shop. It read: *Your past doesn't define you.*

I have kept his card. Sometimes I show it to clients and tell them Kyle's story (protecting his identity, of course).

I hope his story reminds you that you are not defined by the adversities of your past. You can recover. You don't have to be scared.

OWEN: SMALLTOWN BOY

You may remember at the beginning of the book that my own therapy inspired me to become a therapist. It seems fair that I share a little more about that. The final case study is mine.

Some models of therapy actively discourage therapists from sharing their stories with clients. I understand the thinking behind this as the focus should always be on the client. But I also believe that a client needs to know they are in the presence of another human being who understands struggle. Sometimes that involves a degree of self-exposure. If I am asking someone to share their deepest, darkest secrets with me, I feel I owe it to them to reveal some of my own humanity. I follow the same principle with this book. I am sharing how therapy can help you. I could use hundreds of examples of clients I have worked with but I also have to give something of myself. It is my duty and responsibility to practice what I preach.

Therapy for me really was a journey to self-acceptance. I described earlier in the book my first therapy session. I thought I was fine. I wasn't. Therapy taught me that I was filled with shame and that I hadn't accepted my sexuality. I was anxious. I was frightened of taking risks in my life. I wasn't comfortable in my own skin.

This all became clear when I told my story in therapy and then tried to make sense of it. A combination of experiences contributed to my struggles. Witnessing a lot of sectarian violence in Northern Ireland during The Troubles was one. Growing up gay in a Catholic culture of judgement and shame was another. And there was the bullying and rejection during my school years, plus a host of other adverse life events.

Consequently, I didn't feel safe, I didn't feel good enough, I didn't fit in and I didn't know how to be me. But therapy helped me understand why I felt this way, even though my school days were behind me. It saved me.

I learnt not to give myself a hard time. These experiences in my life had happened to me but they didn't define me. Once I understood that, I realised I could work on my negative patterns. I discovered that self-doubt, anxiety and struggle could be turned around. The techniques I have shared with you have been my way through. They still play an active part in my life today.

Despite the impact of negative experiences on my life, I realised that treating myself well and changing my mindset could reverse the effect of those experiences. This was a powerful revelation. That is the power of therapy. You don't have to be a victim of your past.

One of my favourite songs is 'Smalltown Boy' by Bronski Beat. The lyrics tell a story very similar to my own. At points in my life, I too had ran away or turned away. But therapy took me in a different direction. I stopped running away. I faced my story bravely, learnt to celebrate it even, and transformed my life.

I refuse to let my past struggles define me. But I will use them to support my work as a therapist, writer and speaker. This is one of the ways that I've been able to salvage something wonderful from the wreckage of darker times.

I now live my life practising what I have passed on to you in this book. Living this way keeps me grounded, focused and hopeful for the future.

Sometimes I fall and get it wrong. I get up again.

Sometimes I make mistakes. That's OK. I learn from them.

Sometimes I get a little lost. I find my way back.

I hope you find you can do the same. This book can be your roadmap, keeping you on the straight and narrow. It can help you find your way back.

Remember that you never have to stay physically, mentally or emotionally in places that are not healthy for you. Sometimes you may need to physically get away from somewhere, but don't run away from what's going on inside you. Face it all. Let it teach you. Then take the best steps for you.

TIME TO SAY GOODBYE

I must confess, I'm not a fan of goodbyes. I find them difficult. They make me sad. I previously avoided them.

I now know they are important. They honour an experience. They add a sense of completion. They enable moving forward. They close a chapter. They open new chapters.

This is my third book and what I've learnt is that writing self-help books is an illuminating experience. Each time I sit down to write, I imagine I am speaking directly to the reader. Sometimes readers send me messages telling me that my books have changed their lives. And that feedback is life-changing for me, too. I love feeling that synergy with readers.

With that in mind, I want to say goodbye and thank you.

Thank you for reading this book and trusting my experience and this process. Facing your story truthfully will lead you to freedom. Learning to navigate your mind, emotions and behaviours will empower you.

Goodbye for now and hello to a future of new possibilities.

If you would like to find out more about my work, please see:

Instagram and Twitter @owenokaneten
Website: www.owenokane.com
Other books: *Ten to Zen, Ten Times Happier*

USEFUL CONTACT INFORMATION

US MENTAL HEALTH CHARITIES:

https://www.mhanational.org/

https://www.nimh.nih.gov/

https://www.nami.org/Home

https://afsp.org/

https://www.thetrevorproject.org/

https://www.dbsalliance.org/

https://www.activeminds.org/

https://jedfoundation.org/

https://iocdf.org/

Abuse:

https://kathyslegacy.org/

https://www.lifewire.org/about/

https://ncadv.org/about-us

https://preventchildabuse.org/

Addiction:

https://www.shatterproof.org/

https://www.aa.org/

https://www.na.org/

Alzheimer's:

https://www.alz.org/

Grief:

https://copefoundation.org/

Crime:

https://victimsofcrime.org/

https://www.rainn.org/

Eating Disorders:

https://www.nationaleatingdisorders.org/

Learning difficulties:

https://childmind.org/

CANADIAN MENTAL HEALTH CHARITIES:

https://kidshelpphone.ca/

https://www.mhrc.ca/

https://cmha.ca/

https://www.camh.ca/

https://jack.org/Home

https://truenorthaid.ca/northern-health-initiatives/

https://ymhconference.ca/

https://blackhealthalliance.ca/

https://www.youthline.ca/

Abuse:

https://www.prevnet.ca/partners/organizations/
canadian-centre-for-abuse-awareness

https://abusehurts.ca/

Victims of crime:

https://sexualassaultsupport.ca/

https://crcvc.ca/

Addiction:

https://www.farcanada.org/

https://www.drugfreekidscanada.org/

Grief:

https://mygrief.ca/

Alzheimer's:

https://alzheimer.ca/en

Eating disorders:

https://nedic.ca/

Learning difficulties:

https://www.ldac-acta.ca/

ACKNOWLEDGEMENTS

I must thank my agent Bev James and her team for their continued support and enthusiasm. Likewise, the incredible team at my publisher HQ, HarperCollins. I also had the joy of working with Rachel Kenny as my editor again. She is simply brilliant. And to every client who has trusted me with their story, thank you. Everyone else, you know who you are.

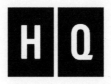

ONE PLACE. MANY STORIES

Bold, innovative and
empowering publishing.

FOLLOW US ON:

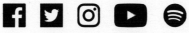

@HQStories